Caregiving – the Inspirational Manual

200 Caregiver Tips with Healthy Lifestyle Benefits

Odell Lendor Glenn Jr.

Kingdom Builders Publications LLC

Caregiving – the Inspirational Manual
Copyright © 2016 by Odell Lendor Glenn, Jr.
Kingdom Builders Publications

All rights reserved. No part of this book may be reproduced or transmitted in any form or by any means without written permission from the author.

ISBN:
Paperback: 978-0-692-63000-6
Special Edition Hard Cover – 978-0-692-63366-3
Library of Congress Control Number 2016932639

Photography – LH "Just Pose" Photography
Cover Designer – LoMar Designs

Editors:
Mike Takieddine
Kingdom Builders Publications Editorial Staff
Donald Lee
Marie James

Printed in USA
Go to these websites:
www.kingdombuilderspublications.com
www.ogcaregiving.com

All Holy Scriptures are taken from the King James Version of the Bible unless otherwise stated.

REVIEWS

"Odell Lendor Glenn Jr. has delivered a rich and all-encompassing book caregivers worldwide can rely on for practical, emotional and spiritual sustenance. Derived from his ministerial duties, his 8-year journey as primary caregiver to his parents, and his academic accomplishments (a doctorate is currently imminent), he has managed, in a masterful triumph, to fuse his personal experience with a continuous stream of caregiver-relevant Holy Scriptures and long-standing philosophical tenets, to produce a solid rendition of a caregiver's 'round-the-clock duties and inspiring advice and compassion" –from an admiring life-time caregiver. **Mike T., Oxford University graduate, London, England**

"The sheer amount of information in this book alone makes it worth the read but the insightful tips push it to another level. The fact Glenn manages to provide so much data combined with hope and reason is astounding. When finished reading, I felt a sense of optimism and love wash over me. He refocuses the mind of the caregiver to care for themselves as well as their loved ones. The relevant prayers woven in throughout the book make this book a standout on any shelf." **Jessica E., Editorial intern, New York, New York**

"With lots of worthy tips, I am inspired by how one can reflect the Godly element of "Care." I am a PhD scholar, live in a broken family and am the eldest of my siblings. I often get dismayed and seek peace. I love the way the author has described to manage so many golden nuggets into one book. It's the best gift to present to my younger siblings. Love it!" **Marryam B., PhD Scholar of Agricultural Entomolgy. Multan, Pakistan**

"When my mom was in my care I wish I had a book so straightforward and clear as this book is. I pray my children will never need the information found in it. But, if they do I have purchased this for them. It is also a good book to just have in your library. I highly recommend it." **Barbara R., Retiree, Lexington, South Carolina**

"Caregiving - the Inspirational Manual by Odell Lendor Glenn Jr. is a must have for all readers. I am only twenty-six years old and I'm still a college student. Recently, my grandparents have not been able to do a lot of things like putting on socks, forgetting to turn the stove off and other things. I have to help them out daily and with a full load of school and now worrying about them, it's hard. However, I found this book to be a perfect guide which basically walked me through everything I needed to know. Odell Lendor Glenn Jr. definitely has helped me in my process of caregiving with my grandparents. I felt so alone, confused, and didn't know much. This book has it all. Tips, suggested activities, advice and much more. Absolutely amazing! Plus, it was inspiring to read this by someone who went through the same thing as I am starting to go through myself. I highly recommend this spectacular book to readers worldwide. No matter what age you find yourself becoming a caregiver, this has all the information you need. I loved it and rate it a five out of five stars." **Danielle U., Full time college student, Little Rock, AR**

"Odell Lendor Glenn Jr's experience and journey will definitely inspire and encourage every caregiver. The tips provided by him are straightforward, sensible and pragmatic and has vividly explained what caregiving brings to daily life. I wish every caregiver should read this book and if you are not a caregiver then this book will guide to develop character, endurance, strength, will and perseverance in your life. If you love and care for someone, the best thing you can do for them is to read this beautiful book." **Dhariyash R., Electrical Engineer, Delft, The Netherlands**

"In the dedication at the beginning of his book, Odell Lendor Glenn Jr. writes, "To my Lord and Savior Jesus Christ: Early in life, I prayed You would 'use me for Your glory'." Glenn has served the Lord well writing a book which is essential reading for anyone who has devoted his or her life to the role of caregiver. Written in a down-to-earth, easy-to-read and engaging style Glenn's 200 tips provide sound advice based on the wisdom of personal experience as a full-time caregiver for both parents (and while completing a doctor in chemical engineering). Glenn is encouraging and inspiring. He provides meaningful prayers and appropriate passages from Holy Scriptures, testimony to his other role as an ordained minister. In additional to the spiritual sustenance Glenn includes helpful advice for a healthier lifestyle including the use of essential oils. The book is a framework for life which must be read by anyone who serves as a caregiver." — **Malcolm N, international journalist and author, San Diego, California**

"Odell Lendor Glenn, Jr.'s book entitled **Caregiving – the Inspirational Manual: 200 Caregiver Tips with Healthy Lifestyle Benefits** offers much-needed practical advice, love, and encouragement to all caregivers who face the daily challenges of caring for the needs of others.

As aging parents become more dependent, the tough reality is someone must step in and offer assistance with daily tasks. Odell took on the job of assisting both his parents. This move posed challenges to both his personal and professional life. Inspired by his faith and his remarkable parents to persevere, Odell did just that. His eye-opening experience led him to write this book to assist other present and future caregivers to find their balance, health, and happiness amid the daily struggles of the job.

One of the great ironies of caregivers is they don't generally take great care of their own health, even though they are available around the clock to assist others.

Mr. Glenn cites a study which claims "More than half (51%) of the caregivers surveyed say they don't have time to take care of themselves, and almost half (49%) said they're too tired to take care of themselves." Odell has included an entire section of tips to help each caregiver develop a healthy lifestyle. He also addresses the necessary legal, financial, and medical roles caregivers play and how to navigate these waters.

As a former caregiver, I urge all caregivers to read this book for its useful information and tips and to remind yourself how incredibly important and unselfish the act of caregiving is.

"To love another person is to see the face of God."
--Victor Hugo, author "Les Miserables"

Kathleen D., Certified Nurse Assistant (CNA)-Grants Pass, Oregon

Odell Lendor Glenn, Jr.

This Book Belongs to

CONTENTS

	REVIEWS	iii
	THE AUTHOR'S DEDICATION	x
	AN OPENING PRAYER FOR CAREGIVERS	xii
1	IN HONOR OF MY PARENTS	13
2	CAREGIVING OVERVIEW	18
3	CAREGIVER CHARACTERISTICS	26
4	TYPICAL PRIMARY CAREGIVER DUTIES	30
5	QUALITY MOMENTS BETWEEN CAREGIVER AND CARE RECIPIENT	35
6	SUGGESTED CAREGIVER ACTIVITIES	38
7	TAKING PICTURES	44
8	DOCTOR/NURSE INTERACTION	47
9	EXTENDED FAMILY SUPPORT	50
10	HOUSEKEEPING	53
11	CARE FOR THE CAREGIVER	60
12	SOCIAL ADVICE	68
13	HEALTHY EATING	73
14	ESSENTIAL OIL BENEFITS	81
15	WHAT "NOT"TO DO AS A CAREGIVER	90
16	BIBLICAL/PHILOSPHICAL PRINCPLES	94
17	CAREGIVER REWARDS	108
18	REFERENCES	116
19	SPECIAL THANKS	122
20	ABOUT THE AUTHOR	125

THE AUTHOR'S DEDICATION

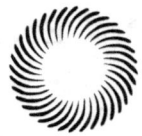

To my Lord and Savior Jesus Christ:

I will never forget the tender age of 10, when You and I had an encounter at a baptismal service. The memory is still very much vivid in my mind. Since then, my faith has developed and You have both directed and guided my footsteps every step of the way. Thank You for Your wisdom and guidance. I love my life with You. I want for nothing with You. I love You with my heart, soul and mind. You are with me everywhere I go and You are my everything. When I take a look back on some of the roads I have traveled, very few are on them, however You continue to provide me with Your grace and wisdom. Early in life, I prayed You would "use me for Your glory." You are doing just that and I'm grateful. I feel as if I soar high like an eagle with You. Walking with You along this journey has made the road an adventure. I am never alone with You. You continue to stretch my faith. If the future looks any brighter, I may need to wear permanent sunglasses! Love You for the many sides of You I get to share with You!

I am honored to serve you beloved; Odell Lendor Glenn Sr. and Sara Vermae Ables-Glenn. Both of you are "royal diadem." The glory of God perpetually rests on the two of you.

I love you Mom and Dad. You have constantly been there for me and most importantly, have consistently understood my unique gifts I have and continue to bring to this world. I am grateful and honored to be named after you. Thank you for attending each graduation, each ordination, each athletic event and allowing me to be free. I count it all joy to daily serve you. Other than my Savior, Himself, there is no one else whom love and understand me more than you two. I now know I am "on

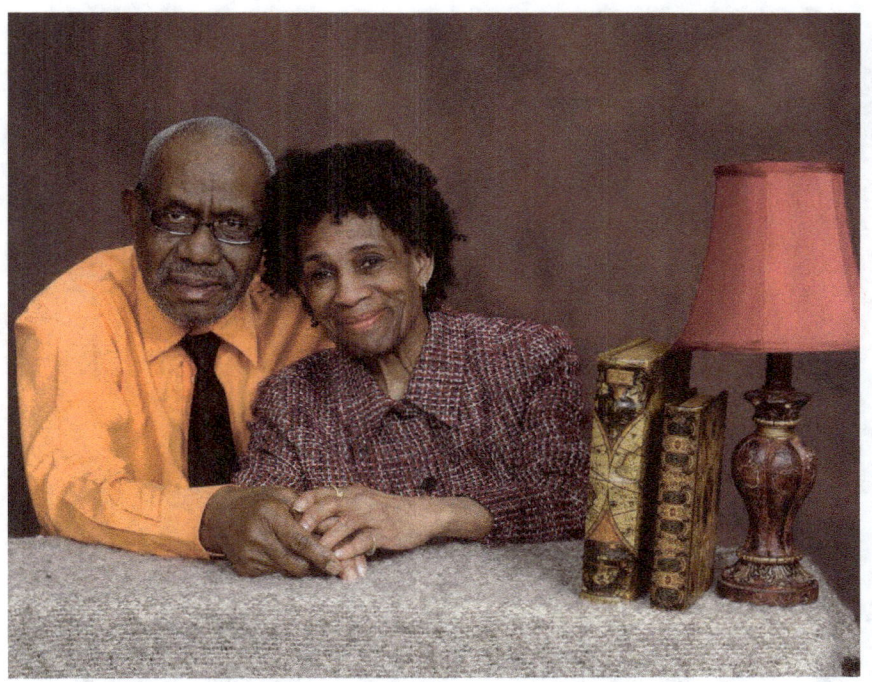

divine assignment" to assist you in this stage of your lives. I am trusting God through and along the process. I am expecting my days here on planet earth to be long and prosperous as the Holy Scripture promises me.

This book is also dedicated to my sister, the late Miss Odette Linda Glenn. Months before you transitioned, you gave me hints I would be the one to help Mom and Dad through the next phase of their journey. Having lived across the street from them in a brownstone in Brooklyn, New York, you kept your eye on them in their very early years of retirement.

I have never forgotten the ornament you purchased for me saying, "THINK BIG." It was the best gift!! I cherish those words and they are implanted in my spirit. To this day, I have never stopped believing and acting on those words. Your spirit still lives with the family. Rest in peace, until we meet again on the other side.

AN OPENING PRAYER FOR CAREGIVERS

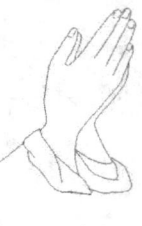

Often overlooked, unnoticed, misunderstood and underappreciated, however, according to Proverbs 15:3, "Your eyes are in every place, beholding both the evil and the good." We continually thank You for the wisdom, grace and strength that You faithfully give us each day. We thank You for stretching our faith and strengthening our trust in You throughout each endeavor. Lord, we ask that You would touch our loved ones and give them peace in the midst of challenge. We know that You can do all things but fail. Continue to lead us and guide us as our hearts reflect You through selfless service and giving. In Jesus' name. AMEN.

IN HONOR OF MY PARENTS

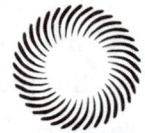

Odell Lendor Glenn, Sr., my Dad, born September 27, 1933, in the small town of Ward, South Carolina. He is the youngest male child of nine children born to the late Berry Glenn Sr. and Bernice Campbell-Glenn.

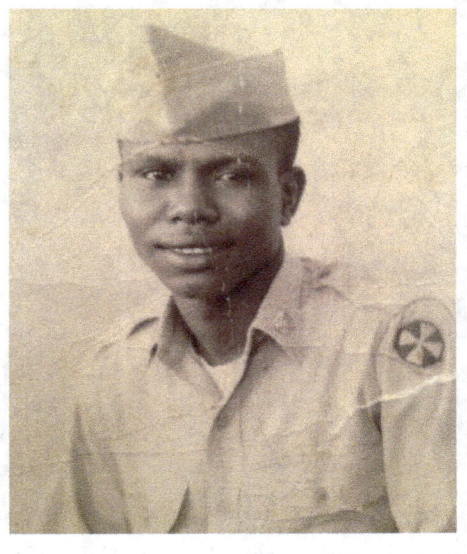

Sara Vermae Ables-Glenn, my Mom, born on July 25, 1934 in Ridge Spring, South Carolina to the late Willie and Rosa Hopkins-Ables. She is the youngest of 5 children.

During Dad's high school years, he was a star basketball player at Ridge Hill High School in Ridge Spring, South Carolina, and he was noted for scoring countless points for team wins. It was at Ridge Hill High School where he met his sweetheart and present wife for over 60 years, Sara Ables. Odell Glenn graduated from Ridge Hill High School on May 21, 1952 and, one year later, he married Sara Ables-Glenn on May 30, 1953.

Glenn enlisted into the U.S. Armed forces and served in the Korean War under President Harry Truman. The Korean War occurred over a conflict between the U.S. and the Soviet Union with regard to Korea. President Truman issued an executive order to integrate the military two years before the war started, but many senior commanders ignored this command.

Dad described numerous stories on how he saw soldiers killed around him, not to mention the endless bloodshed of innocent victims. He would also reflect on the racial tensions which occurred between he and his white counterparts during those times. He recalled knowing how the prayers of his father, Berry Glenn, provided him with continuous support.

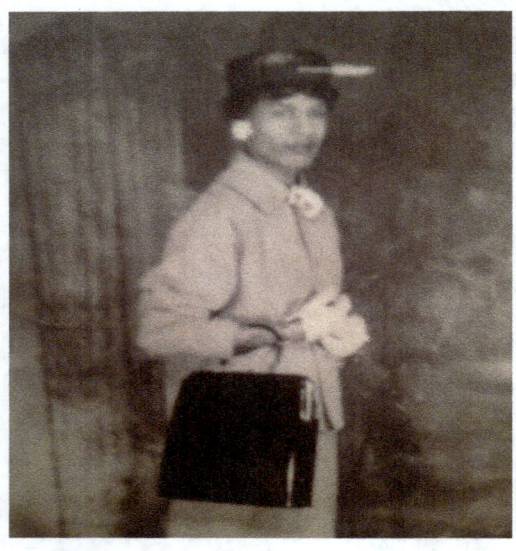

Dad never failed to thank God for sparing his life throughout the war and received four honorable medals for his services. These included "The National Defense Service Medal", "The Korean Service Medal", "The United Nations Service Medal", and "The Good Conduct Medal." While he was in the army, Mom worked in the school system with her sister, the late Thelma Ables-Coleman.

When the war ended, Dad returned to South Carolina and worked for a year as a porter with E.I. DuPont Company in Aiken, South Carolina. A year later, in 1956, he and his family moved to Brooklyn, New York. He continued to work as a chef in various restaurants in Manhattan of which, notably, were several elite Italian restaurants in the heart of NYC. He later worked as a chauffeur for the Long Island Railroad for 20 years until he retired on August 1, 1997.

Mom had various jobs as a cashier in New York City at places such as Macy's and Goodwin's department stores. She also served as a tour guide at the World's Center Park in Queens, New York. She attended both Queens College and Brooklyn College and picked up early childhood development college credit. She later worked as a day care teacher in Brooklyn, New York until she retired in 1999. While working at the day care center, Mom was well known for her kindness, and her students adored her. To this day, many of her former students have gone on to graduate from medical or law school and still remain fond of those earlier memories.

Mom was also noted for being a church decorator. She was depended upon to decorate the church around special holidays such as Christmas, Resurrection Sunday and special programs. Her creativity and artistic attributes delighted many parishioners. Her home continues to be a model reminder of her special talent and creative attributes. Another talent she enjoyed was acting. She loved to dress up in costumes and act in inspirational plays. She was also very fond of African attire and impressed many with her unique gift of accessories to complement what she would wear.

In addition, both of them continue to serve as role models and mentors, as well as parental figureheads to our youth and young adults. Many old acquaintances to this day still call my parents "pa" and "ma."

Dad and Mom were both proud owners of a home in Brooklyn with a two-car garage, a basketball court and several guest rooms. It was a rare and distinguished privilege to own a home, as there were not a plethora of them in the Bedford Stuyvesant area. At one point, Mom and Dad took in other children to come in live with them and family members from the south and north stayed at the home for extended periods of time. Some came for permanent relocation purposes or for short- term employment opportunities in NYC. Others came simply for pleasure. Whatever their reasons were for an extended stay, they were always received with open arms.

In the community, Dad alternated as treasurer and vice president of the block association throughout the years. Several block association meetings were held at my parents' home. Whenever block parties were held during the summer, Mom and

Dad managed to provide everyone on the block (including friends of friends) with food and entertainment. They made their home a place where everyone could feel comfortable. Mom assisted Dad in the community by working alongside him in all his capacities. She turned the home into a comfort zone in which people could drop their guard and simply relax to their hospitality. They had a listening ear and warm advice. Their compassion, warm spirit and humble demeanor, then and to this day, enriched people's lives and endowed them with a serene sense of love, freedom and happiness.

Dad and Mom had four children of their own. They had two girls and then waited ten years to have the two boys. Out of these blessings came a wonderful son-in-law, two wonderful granddaughters and two great grandchildren.

After living in Brooklyn for over 50 years, Mom and Dad relocated to the south and purchased a home in a cul-de-sac community in South Carolina. They remained active in the Senior citizens' community, and in church. They worship and serve with their son and caregiver, the Reverend Odell Glenn Jr., while other siblings and best friends still live within the vicinity. This joyful phenomenon is portrayed throughout the book. Needless to say, both parents have lived –and continue to live- fruitful lives full of blessings.

Dear Readers,

Caregiving is indeed a challenging undertaking, one which honors me each and every day as I serve as primary caregiver to my parents. The debt of love I owe is priceless.

This book is intended to share wisdom I've gained and inform other kind and gracious folk. It is primarily intended for those current caregivers and others who are uncertain about the roles they might play, and what daily caregiving entails. Further, it serves as a general self-help manual providing guidelines and inspirational talk to caregivers. It also has chapters devoted to healthy eating lifestyles (as well as the benefits of essential oils) which in my opinion -and of the experts- contain hefty benefits for care recipients. Although the foundational attitudes and tasks of caregiving remain constant, people will surely have their own unique experiences. Provided are prayers I personally reflect upon as a caregiver which can be very useful.

For those of you who would like to read beyond these pages, references and source articles are included at the end of the book.

I am available to come to your city, country, church, workshop, non-profit organization, institution, educational facility, group discussion, business, etc. for group discussions and book signings regarding my **"Caregiving –the Inspirational Manual" and 200 tips**.

CAREGIVING OVERVIEW

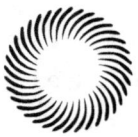

TIP #1

Today, people are generally more health conscious in terms of their lifestyles, particularly with food and exercise. This naturally reflects in part on why more people are living beyond 70 years of age. Adult children are now left in a position where they have to take on the role of caregivers for aging parents –many find themselves in the precarious predicament of having to look after both the generations of their children as well as their parents. Research refers to this as "the sandwich generation", and we should expect this trend to rise steadily. If you find yourself having to adjust to suddenly providing daily care to your loved ones, do not panic, you are not alone.

TIP #2

According to the Journal of Aging and Social Policy, (2008), there are more than 44 million unpaid caregivers who provide care to people aged 18 and older who are ill, aging or have a disability. You may also find yourself with little to no income while you provide the care. What some of us could do, if at all possible, is to try starting a legitimate home based business. Alternatively, some of us may also want to take some online courses to sharpen our skills. Online courses and colleges are on the rise, and there are financial resources available to help pay for them. I would encourage you to seek those courses in line with what you would like to add to your education. Education and learning in general, is something you can never say you've "finished and done with." One should constantly learn and update skills analogous to technology. Ten years from now, make sure you can say you chose your life and did not settle for it. In other words, work around any obstacles. As you grow more, you see more. As you know more you can achieve more.

TIP #3

According to the Gerontological Society of America, adult children are more likely to serve as primary caregivers than any other group. The study showed 41% of adult children served as compared to 38.5% for spouses and 20.4% for other family members. The study also showed more and more caregivers are working alone without secondary backup. Capable siblings are the first to normally show up and share in the responsibility. At early onset of dementia, the task may be easy, but as time goes on, seek out help so you will not be on your own and risk burning out.

TIP #4

Caregivers suffer loss of wages, health insurance, employment benefits, retirement savings, investments, and at times, Social Security benefits. These losses naturally can lead to serious consequences for the long term "career caregiver." Be aware this may happen, especially if it comes to the point where you can no longer work outside of the home. Talk with your employer to see if there are any options. Do not suddenly jump to dire conclusions such as you may not be able to ever work outside of the home. You may suffer financially, but remain creative and productive. *"Do the best you can until you know better. Then, when you know better, do better."* (Maya Angelou)

TIP #5

Surveyed caregivers say the reason they do not go to the doctor is because they put their family's needs first (67%), or they put the care recipient's needs over their own (57%). More than half (51%) said they do not have time to take care of themselves, and almost half (49%) said they are too tired to do so. As a caregiver, you must remember to tend to your own needs. You don't want to depart before the person you are caring for. Balance your life by building down time into your schedule and rethinking your overall responsibilities and errands.

TIP #6

The National Alliance for Caregiving (N.A.C. 2004) reported 73% of surveyed caregivers admit praying helps cope with caregiving stress. I too have a testimony that prayer and Bible reading have benefits. Miracles which cannot be explained have occurred and have strengthened my faith.

> *"Constant in hope, patience in tribulation and instant in prayer."*
> Romans 12:12 (KJV).

In other words, we have a great expectation for a better outcome; knowing that even through trials, patience and consistent prayer will be our help. Praying for others will cause healing in them, ourselves and our loved ones.

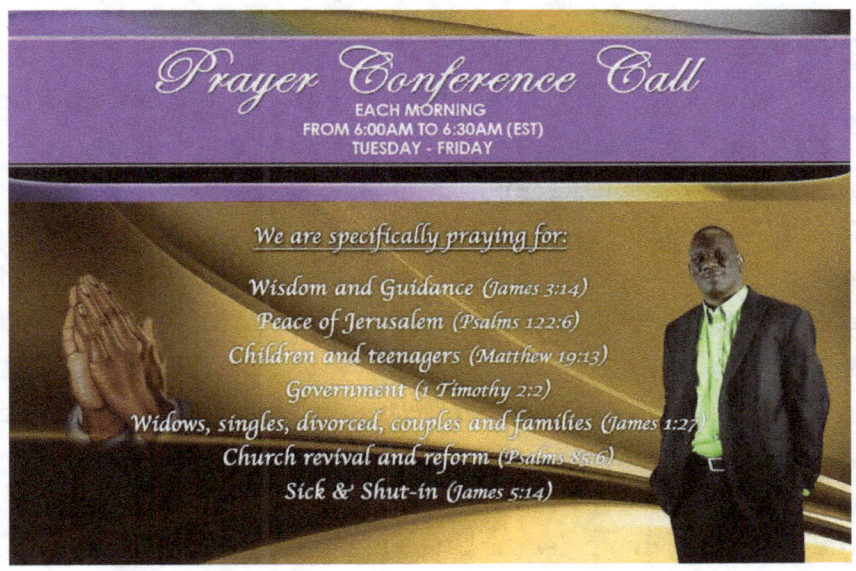

> *"Pray one for another, that ye may be healed."*
> **James 5:16 (KJV).**

Prayer will give you strength, hope, guidance and "direction for the long journey." Continue to ask for wisdom and guidance, and you will look back and witness miracles from simply asking.

TIP #7

According to the National Alliance for Caregiving (N.A.C. 2004), more caregivers are women (61%) than men (39%). Typically, women do the heavy lifting more so than men. Regardless of the gender, ask for help so you may complete the task successfully. The daily task of caregiving will be the same regardless of gender.

TIP #8

Research suggests the number of male caregivers may be increasing and will continue to grow due to a variety of social demographic factors. "Men as Caregivers" (November 2012). Men, you are not alone. As a male, you will at times not only serve as a caregiver, but also act as provider and emotional as well as moral support for the care recipient and their entire family.

After preaching three family funerals, moving from state to state, serving as primary caregiver, minister, and a working professional, I can share from first-hand experience, the lessons I have learned were valuable and numerous. Jogging, walking, journaling, reading, and exercise can be great ways to relieve stress, especially if you are the guru the family depends upon. These things have worked well for me.

TIP #9

More often than not, as a caregiver, the roles get reversed. Don't be surprised if it seems like you become the parent to the care recipient. Alzheimer's is a type of dementia which causes problems with memory, thinking, and behavior. It is not a part of normal aging. It worsens over time, and it currently has no cure. It degrades the adult parent to behave like a child and in some cases, it causes them to be worse than a child.

You may find yourself being more of the parent when the disease worsens. The roles get reversed without your ever wanting or having to become the parent. Make sure you know what a "power of attorney" is and where to go and get one. You will find yourself constantly protecting and planning each day for your loved one. Read books on how to care for someone with this type of disease. There are lots of "dementia training classes" now available.

TIP #10

In-home elder care is an alternative to a nursing home or assisted living care facility. Seniors tend to respond best to in-home care with a family member. They adapt and become familiar in the comfort of their own homes. For as long as you can keep your loved one in the home, keep them there.

I was able to keep my loved one in the home with me for 8 years. Dad still remembers me and tells me in many ways how he appreciates the things I have done and still do. In the midst of the challenges, they still remember who loves them and what they do. Never forget that!!

TIP #11

Care recipients deserve no less than the best caregivers have to offer. Unless you are a caregiver, 99.9% of people can never figure out how you manage to put on that smile each and every day, nor how you keep giving the best you have to give. How you make others feel about themselves says a lot about you.

CAREGIVING OVERVIEW PRAYER

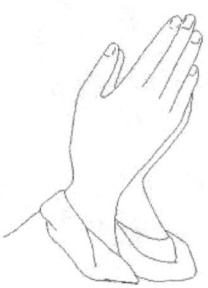

We thank You for research facts that help keep us aware of what may we encounter as we age. However, we trust You to guide us through the process and we thank You for your faithfulness that has never left us and will never leave us. As we walk by faith and not by sight, we trust that You provide us with the wisdom and grace that would lead us on. Your Word tells us in Psalms 37:8, You will instruct us and teach us in the way we shall go. We are encouraged that You will guide us with Your eyes. We claim victory through faith that You will see us through and that all of our needs will be met according to Your riches and glory. In Jesus' name. Amen.

CAREGIVER CHARACTERISTICS

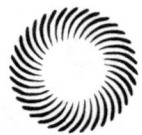

TIP #12

Daily caregiving is a test which measures character, strength, perseverance, will and endurance. Caregiving also requires patience. If you do not have patience, you will not be an effective caregiver.

TIP #13

Caregiving is a divine calling. Everyone is not suited for full time caregiving duty. Accept this fact.

TIP #14

When the family begins to search for the right candidate or candidates for caregiving (if it has not already come naturally to the care recipient), make sure the appointed caregiver has endurance for the journey. Look for the person or people who are not selfish and has a willingness to serve daily.

TIP #15

If you are an only child, you may not have a choice in the matter. Seek help immediately if you do not have the time and the patience. Caregivers must be able to sustain themselves over the long journey.

TIP #16

Persons who do not like the sight of hospitals, and who tend to make decisions hastily or based on emotions are not suitable for the arduous tasks of caregiving.

TIP #17

Caregivers must be versatile in terms of their schedule. Each day may be different with new or altered problems to solve in unplanned time frames. If you are a routine-type person, the job will not be suitable for you. You must be able to adapt to the need at hand.

TIP #18

Caregiving is all about personality. The questions you must ask yourself are "How does my personality fit with what my care recipient needs? Can I care for the care recipient with my character traits? Do our personalities clash?

TIP #19

Caregivers are like engineers because they are problem solvers. From sunrise to sunset, the caregiver is strategizing and searching for the optimal model best suited for the patient. Each day is a quest to keep the patient healthy and stimulated and should bring something new that could be dealt with. For example, there are times when the caregiver will have to interface with the medical team (primary physician, visiting nurses, and other), or with family members, to resolve issues on the patient's behalf and wellbeing. There is hardly a dull day while on a caregiving mission.

TIP #20

Self-criticism is part of the caregiving mission. Admit your mistakes and move on. If you cannot admit mishaps then you are not a good fit. Be open to change and new ways of doing things.

TIP #21

Caregivers pass on good moral practices to family and friends. They serve as models. You become a role model for generations to come in the event something would ever happen not only to yourself but to other family members when they get older. Assume the role model as best you can, for it will keep your morale and self-esteem uplifted.

CAREGIVING CHARACTERISTICS PRAYER

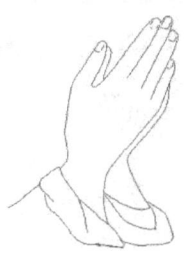

Touch those caregivers who are the only child. Lord, grace them with knowledge and strength for the long road ahead of them. Send angels to help them and give them rest. Bless families that have more than one person capable of caregiving. Allow the families to work together to relieve the stress of one person. We rebuke excuses. Give them the wisdom to work together and put aside differences. And for that one person or persons who steps up to the challenge, shower them with Your blessings. You remind us that You are eternal God and our refuge. Your arms are everlasting and we have comfort in knowing that we are safe and secure underneath them. And so we put our small hands into Your great big hands. Lead us and guide us in all we do. In Jesus' name. Amen.

TYPICAL PRIMARY CAREGIVER DUTIES

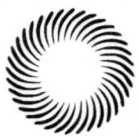

TIP #22

The job of a primary caregiver is hard work especially if you are caring for the patient at home. If it had been an easy, everyone would be doing it. It can vary from person to person and from need to need. I like to compare it to a corporate career in terms of three levels of management: Executive, mid-level and entry-level management. Live-in caregivers work amongst these 3 levels 24 hours a day, 7 days a week. Even if you are employed outside of the home, your subconscious is permanently aware of your caregiving duties at home. You learn to adjust accordingly.

TIP #23

Executive management may involve things like administering medication and making sure medications are taken each day at the correct time. Part of this includes the more general planning for the week/month, planning trips, managing finances, budgeting, paying bills, strategizing, providing emotional support, and preparing for errands and expenses. Your own needs constantly become secondary.

TIP #24

Mid-level management is made up of hands-on patient care practices. This includes both integration and interaction with doctors, nurses, caregiving agencies, associations and support groups. You serve as a liaison between the doctor and the patient by identifying changes in the patient's condition, and then reporting symptoms to the medical team who supports the patient. Your job also includes keeping up with doctor appointments for the one or more patients you care for. You may be the deciding factor whether or not prescribed medications work for your patient, then report this information to the primary doctor.

TIP #25

Entry-level management is not menial work. It includes hands-on work which must get done. This includes: bathing, grooming, hair, finger, and toenail care, brushing, oral care and other personal care. Food preparation will range from grocery shopping to actually preparing the food. Also included are housecleaning, transferring the care recipient from chairs, toilet, in and out of bed, and to and from an automobile. It involves the purchase of canes, walkers, wheelchairs and ramps. You may be the only source of transportation they have, which means personal car maintenance becomes very important.

TIP #26

The most important out of all of these management styles is the companionship and emotional support you give the care recipient on a daily basis. It is up to you to bring a smile to the patient's face and keep them stimulated and feeling safe.

TIP #27

Companionship entails gentle conversation and indulging in joint activities including reading the Bible, watching TV, playing card games, undertaking tasks in the yard when the weather is nice, and escorting the care recipient out, when their condition permits, to church, to the mall and wherever else the care recipient enjoys.

TIP #28

No two care recipients are alike, and no caregiving styles and job duties are the same. Some care recipients suffer from memory loss while others are sharp and coherent. Some struggle to get around while others do not. When it comes to daily caregiving, it is important to keep in mind duties will vary and you have to be able to adapt and respond to each care recipient individually.

When you have done all you can do to keep your loved one in the home, and the time has come to move on, you can feel confident that highly qualified health care professionals will look after your loved one in an extended care facility, particularly when you visit your loved one as frequently as your circumstances permit. My prayer is that God gives you both grace and strength to do all you can possibly do.

TIP #29

You will find yourself constantly planning for the next hour, the next day, the next week, the next month, the next season, and the next year for each individual care recipient. As men, we tend not to ask for help. Don't wait until a crisis occurs to reach out for support. As my Dad's illness worsened, I had no choice but to have early morning and late afternoon home care assistance come in my home and give me a helping hand.

TIP #30

If you are a male caregiver, don't be surprised if you find yourself purchasing a bra for mom at a "Victoria's Secret" clothing store or negotiating a hairstyle with the beauty parlor stylist. When you are the primary caregiver, you have to handle it all, even when it isn't seemly.

TIP #31

While mom is getting her nails and feet done, as a male caregiver, you and Dad may be the only two males in the parlor, perhaps also getting yours done.

CAREGIVING DUTIES PRAYER

The daily tasks sometimes seem more than normal and so we ask You for daily strength. You made us human and so we have finite capacity. However, You are infinite in both power and strength. Equip us to hear Your voice and guide us through the journey. Set up divine connections that would make the path a little less cumbersome. We admit, at times we feel lonely and helpless but help us to know You are with us every step of the way. We want dearly to see our loved ones whole, but You have a plan greater than our thoughts. We thank You for the comfort in knowing You will never leave us nor will You forsake us. Thank You in advance. In Jesus' name. Amen.

QUALITY MOMENTS BETWEEN CAREGIVER AND CARE RECIPIENT

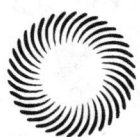

TIP #32

Church attendance, activities, and programs are very important, especially if they previously had positions and were very active. Sign them up for celebrations and programs which either you or someone else is involved. Keep them learning and doing!

TIP #33

Find out what activities they loved doing and hone in on them. Invite the family and friends to visit or to phone and talk to the care recipient.

TIP #34

Bring back memories through a discussion of past events. Visits with first cousins and old classmates are pleasant moments. Dad was blessed to have a best friend since high school. Saturday morning visits can bring tears of joy to their eyes and yours.

TIP #35

When having quality time with the care recipient, find a place relatively quiet. The surroundings should support the person's ability to focus on his or her thoughts.

The best portions of life with the care recipient will be those small, nameless moments you spend smiling and listening.

QUALITY MOMENT PRAYER

There is indeed a time for everything underneath the sun. A time to dance and a time to rejoice. While we have those precious moments, help us to make the best of them. **Ecclesiastes 3:1** tells us "To everything there is a season, and a time to every purpose under the heaven." Thank You for blessed assurance in knowing while we quietly and daily give care, You will give us peace in our spirits. Help us to appreciate the value on time and treat it similar to a precious commodity. We thank You for every moment of it. In Jesus' name. AMEN.

SUGGESTED CAREGIVER ACTIVITIES

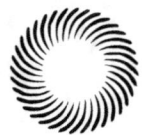

TIP #36

Instead of driving long distances, try taking the train (AMTRAK) or bus (Megabus) services. You will be amazed at how relaxing the trip can be. You can get work done on your laptop or tablet, and your loved one or care recipient might even strike up a conversation or friendship with someone else.

TIP #37

Take loved ones on trips that nurture relaxation. You may not get all of the free time you want, but the trip will do both you and them good overall.

TIP #38

Keep your loved one with other people, and as actively involved as you can during the holidays.

TIP #39

Keep them involved in your neighborhood community center for seniors. My parents happened to be the "king" and "queen" in 2012. Your local senior community center has ongoing activities such as exercise, current event information and picnics and lunch for your loved ones. Some centers will actually pick them up and bring them back home while you are employed outside of the home.

TIP #40

Be abreast of holidays such as Black History month and Valentine's Day in February. Remind them of holidays and have them dress up for the occasion.

TIP #41

If at all possible, take your loved ones to football games to volunteer their time. According to research, individuals who volunteer may live longer than people who do not give up some of their time. In the southern part of the United States, college football teams are an integral part of the culture. Involve them in it. I have taken Mom to the University of South Carolina's football games to volunteer at concession stands via a church function and she loved it. Annual state fairs are another great social outlet.

TIP #42

During winter months, mall visits can be a time to exercise through walk. Mall walks can also be a time for them to reflect, relax, and meet new people.

TIP #43

Local high school football games (August - November) are exciting as well. In our case, our local high school happened to be directly across from our cul-de-sac (gated community). Events such as these have saved me time and gas in terms of long distance driving to and from games.

TIP #44

Keeping your loved ones active in church with you could result in rewards later on. Mom was honored as "MOTHER OF THE YEAR." Dad was honored as "FATHER OF THE YEAR." I, as caregiver, was one proud son! Gifts, money, prizes and trips were given on their behalf. It's great to be and feel appreciated.

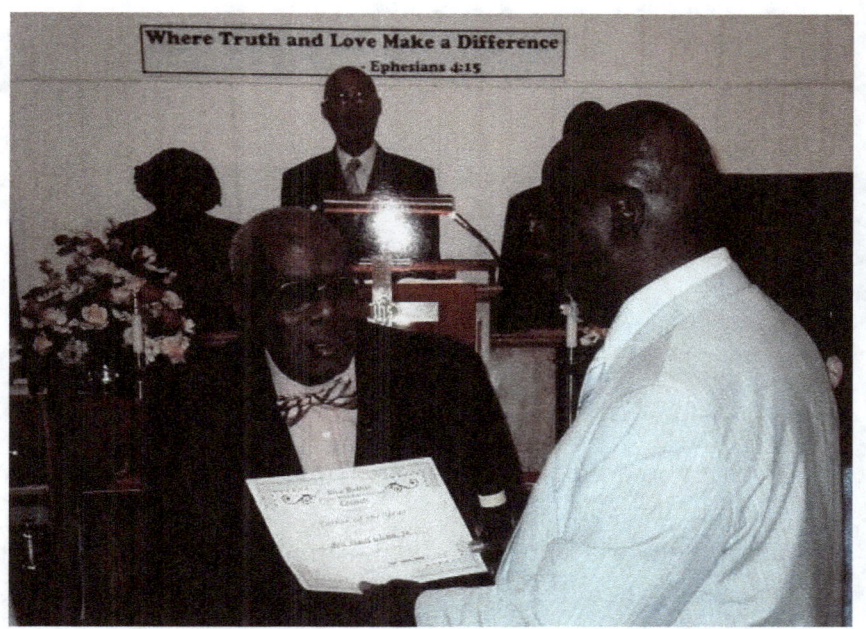

TIP #45

Family is not defined only as blood relatives. They are also the people in your life who want you in their lives. They are the ones who would do anything to see you smile and who love you no matter what. I am reminded of the Holy Scripture in **Matthew 12:50 (KJV)** where Jesus says *"For whosoever shall do the will of my Father which is in Heaven, the same is my brother, and sister, and mother."*

TIP # 46

Quality time with old friends brings back precious memories. If at all possible, value those hours with them. Reviving old times are valuable moments.

TIP #47

Even if you are not a church goer or affiliated with any church or community outreach facility, or if you do not have a large family to network with, keep them active in social events. Listen to what and where they might want to go and do it on a weekly basis. You will learn a lot.

For example, Mom developed a passion while living in the south for *"Strawberry Picking."* She loves to attend events like this. Also, keep them abreast on current events and what happens politically and socially around them.

SUGGESTED ACTIVITIES PRAYER

*The earth is the Lord's, and the fullness thereof; the world, and they that dwell therein. **(Psalms 24:1 KJV)** We thank You for abundant life. We thank You for places to go, sights to see and events to attend with our loved ones. Whether or not it is to a mall, a football game, an ice cream parlor, a church service, a movie or a trip out of town, protect us as we go to and fro. Bless our going out and our coming in. Protect us on the highways within automobiles, airplanes, trains and buses. As we plan for trips, we want Your presence to lead and guide us everywhere we go. Thank You in advance for using us as vessels in service. In Jesus' name. AMEN.*

TAKING PICTURES

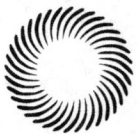

TIP #48

Take plenty of pictures of you and your loved ones or care recipients together. This should include professional pictures taken in and around the home, outside amongst the community, during the holiday seasons and with other family members. Keep a journal through pictures. You will cherish those moments in years to come.

TIP #49

Take time to organize family photo albums as well as making honors, plaques and awards visible. Someone has to do it. You are called the "caregiver" because you "care."

TIP #50

Make sure they are involved in their grandchildren's and great grandchildren's lives. They love grandchildren and speak of them often.

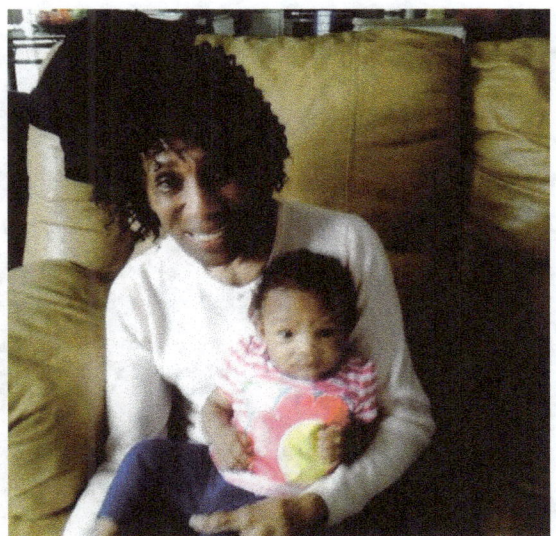

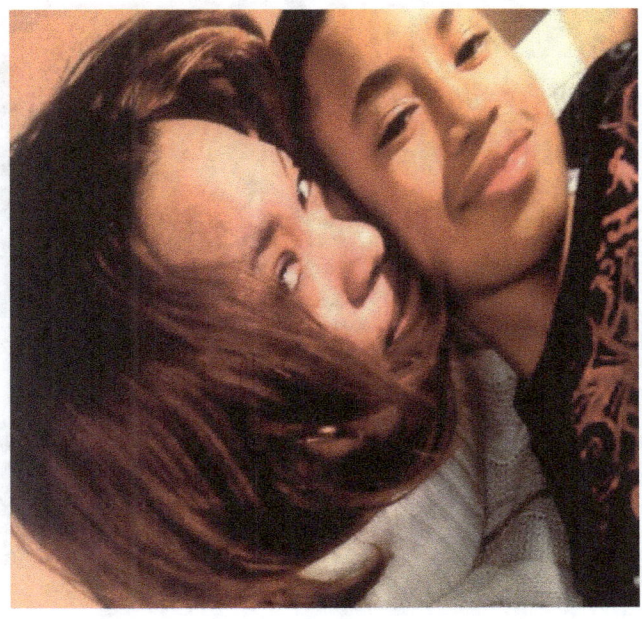

TAKING PICTURES PRAYER

We thank You for technological advances that allow us to take photos of places and family and then share them with each other. We display the glory of God through capturing a moment in time with a photograph. Psalms 104:31 tells us "May the glory of the Lord endure forever; may the Lord rejoice in His works." Ephesians 2:10 reminds us "For we are His workmanship, created in Christ Jesus for good works, which God prepared beforehand, that we should walk in them." Whenever and wherever we are, help us not to forget that a photo is memorable and will last a lifetime. Help us to be sensitive to both time and place. Allow our photo albums and digital cameras to tell a story for many generations to come. Allow generations upon generations to witness Your glory. In Jesus' name. AMEN.

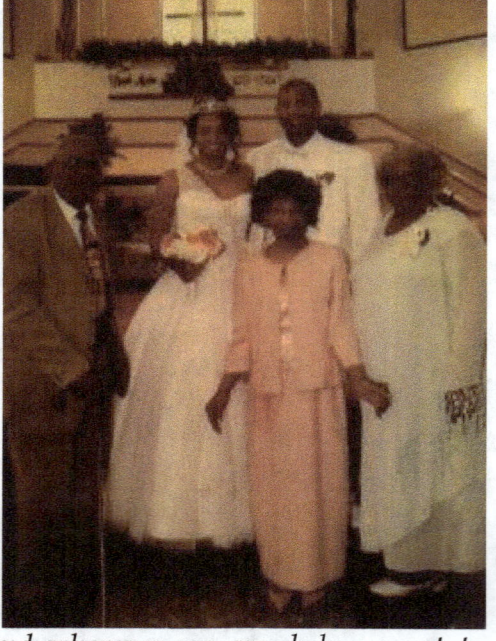

DOCTOR/NURSE INTERACTION

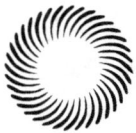

TIP #51

Get to know each doctor on a first name basis. Keep abreast of appointment times and work around your own schedule. They are flexible. Discuss ideas on what you can do at home to make better health choices.

TIP #52

If there is no known cure for the loved one's disease, keep up to date on the latest research. Call, write and/or e-mail your local, state and federal legislators. Let them know how much you would appreciate if more research could be done for your loved one's ailment. Also, inform them that any additional support emotional and financial would help you tremendously with caregiving. March in Washington, D.C. as well as in your local state. Join an organization related to the illness and believe, hope, trust and pray.

TIP #53

Keep a copy of doctor's, nurse's and physician's name and phone number as well as any other important documents in a safe place. Nurses and doctors change locations frequently and/or retire, but for whatever reason, note each name and date each visit. Falls and broken bones can occur as your loved ones age. Make adjustments around the home as needed. Be a team player with the doctor and his or her staff and keep a journal on the day by day progress.

PHYSCIAN'S PRAYER

You are the God our Healer. We thank You for doctors, nurses, physicians and the entire staff at hospitals across the nation. Thank You for the wisdom and knowledge that You have provided them to help us. We ask that You would bless each one. It is Your desire for us to "pray without ceasing." And we continue to pray for cures for diseases and ailments that have no known cure. We ask You to release research funds for more in-depth study on diseases such as Alzheimer's. As we not only pray, but write to senators and march in protest, we are confident that You will answer in your own time. In Jesus' name. AMEN.

EXTENDED FAMILY SUPPORT

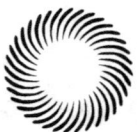

TIP #54

When it came time to relocate from the north to the south, one of the things considered was "proximity to other siblings, children and relatives". Having brothers and sisters together (especially with a small family and after many brothers and sisters have passed on) was a wise choice. Remind family members how grateful you are when they help you out. Don't be afraid to ask for any kind of extra help they can provide.

TIP #55

Annual summer barbecues bring large families together. When planning a major relocation, listen closely to where they want to eventually live while they are still relatively healthy. More often than not, one of them has already told you.

Relocating to where the bulk of both families reside has been beneficial. Going back to where your loved ones grew up will remind them of events, places and people.

TIP #56

Being asked for Thanksgiving Dinner or Christmas Dinner at a sibling's home brings smiles to the loved one. It is always nice when they are asked for fellowship outside their own home.

TIP #57

Time spent with the children's children of your loved one's siblings equally mean a lot to them.

EXTENDED FAMILY PRAYER

Family prayer; a rare deed nowadays. We thank You for family. Remind us of the importance of assembling ourselves together not only during holidays and in time of need, but on a regular basis. Remind us to pray for each other and to be thankful for each other. Bind us together in perfect harmony so that we can number our days that we have together and gain a heart of wisdom. At family reunions, during holiday gatherings, at weddings and graduations and during funerals, allow us to walk into a destiny that pleases You. We ask blessings on family businesses and corporations that the legacy may be handled wisely from generation to generation. We pray that each generation grow closer to You and allow the Holy Spirit to direct and guide. Lamentations 5:19, " For You, O Lord, rule forever, Your throne is from generation to generation." Allow families to remember the covenant You have with them. 1 Chronicles 16:15 "Remember His covenant forever, The word which He commanded to a thousand generations." Allow the legacy on each family to be remembered and known as a praying entity. In Jesus' name. AMEN.

HOUSEKEEPING

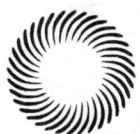

TIP #58

Make sure there is a will in place. If not, get one done ASAP. Make sure the will is registered within your state. Lawyers will not make wills if the loved one is not cognitive enough to understand. Be clear of the loved one's expectations.

There is no way to predict exactly when or where an earthquake or a flood will occur. Seismologists say numerous minor to moderate earthquakes will be felt and major ones are on their way. Flood insurance, earthquake insurance and/or renter's insurance is something we tend to overlook. While you are caring for a loved one at home, it's best to have this and not need it than to need it and not have it. The questions you must consider are:

- Is my home covered if an earthquake or major flood occurs?
- Can I afford the cost of rebuilding or repairing my home if it is damaged due to an earthquake or flood?
- What would it cost to replace my personal belongings?
- How would I pay for temporary housing if damage from an earthquake or flood makes it uninhabitable?

While caring for loved ones, one has to seriously consider all of the consequences.

TIP #59

The power of attorney is a legal document giving someone the power to act and speak on your behalf. In case you ever become mentally incapacitated, you'll need what are known as a *"durable"* power of attorney for medical care and finances. Power of Attorneys can start at $200.00 and up depending on the county and state.

TIP #60

Make sure you fax or mail the power of attorney to each creditor. Not all creditors accept documents via fax. This can be a very grueling process but it is very necessary. This document is highly recommended.

TIP #61

A representative payee is a person, agency, organization or institution you select to manage your funds when determined you are unable to do so yourself. Social Security, in any state, DOES NOT recognize the power of attorney. You have to fill out a representative payee form instead. Read up on this important information at http://www.ssa.gov/payee/.

TIP #62

A health power of attorney allows you to make health decisions on behalf of the individual. This is separate from the normal power of attorney and also entails a separate cost. Make sure you bring this document with you to each doctor visit and to each surgery. Have each doctor's office keep a copy in their office.

TIP #63

This is where you really have to do your homework. Find out the resources available in your state. If you don't look, search, seek, or ask, it can hurt you later on. There is always something out there but you have to be "in the know." In South Carolina, I am able to get a yearly $500.00 voucher from *Central Midland Council of Governments*. It is a yearly respite award program which relieves caregivers. It is certainly not a lot but it helps. Caregiving relief services can cost anywhere from $20.00 to $25.00 an hour. This adds up quickly. Use whatever resources available to you at time of need. Programs tend to change yearly.

TIP #64

If at all possible, have a very serious conversation about your loved one's health wishes. It is NEVER too early to discuss this. You want to know early on whether or not your loved one wants a "DNR" (Do not resuscitate) if they are on life support. The caregiver needs to know this or else you are left to make dreadful decisions on your own in distress. Distress you want to avoid early on and at all cost. Keep abreast of this information before it becomes too late. Whether or not the family decides on a DNR or not, keep a copy visible in the home so if paramedics have to come inside the home they can see official documentation and proceed accordingly.

TIP #65

Make sure the funeral parlor have all important documents, insurances, funeral arrangements and program planned. It is wise to plan this early. This takes a lot of pressure off of you when the time comes. If your loved one has already told you how this should be done, it will make your job easier.

TIP #66

Take the time and energy to research your family history. Know what each person passed away from and the possible causes. Find out what you can do differently. Do your own research and homework. Don't allow the medical doctor to do this for you. Also, seek a second opinion.

TIP #67

If you are married, get to know the family history of your life partner. It will help you be a more effective caregiver.

TIP #68

Trust your instincts. Remember, you know your family member best. Don't ignore what doctors and specialists tell you, but listen to your intuition as well. Don't make decisions based on emotion.

TIP #69

Make sure the caregiving agency is BOTH licensed and bonded. You may have to pay a little more than you normally would for a private caregiver, but it is better to have your loved ones protected from any unforeseen circumstance.

TIP #70

LICENSED means a home care agency is registered to perform certain types of work and only those types of work, such as cleaning, taking loved ones out to the park, etc. As caregiver, you can check up on an agency's current, legal or any other complaints against them. In case of a tragic accident, A BONDED company has secured funds (controlled by the state) available for consumer's claims against the company. This money is directly available to you for various reasons as controlled by a state agency.

TIP #71

If you decide to use a private caregiver because of financial limitations, make sure you thoroughly check the qualifications, paperwork and past performance (references) of the private caregiver. Private caregivers on average cost considerably less than agency caregivers, but you carry a greater burden if they suddenly leave you, or don't show up, or are not working out as you had wanted.

TIP #72

Get to know your next door neighbors as a good point of contact. If you have to go out of town it doesn't hurt to ask your neighbors to keep an eye on your loved ones if they have to stay home alone. Good neighbors will be glad you asked.

TIP #73

If your care recipient is a U.S. veteran, home health care coverage, financial support, nursing home care, and adult day care benefits may be available. Some Veterans Administration programs are free, while others require co-payments, depending upon the veteran's status, income, and other criteria. You have to really do your homework here, so keep up with all receipts and stay on top of this. Make sure they know who you are or else you will slip through the cracks.

TIP #74

Modify the bathrooms, showers and bathroom stools. Ramps outside of the home may also be an additional cost for a loved one who cannot climb stairs. These adjustments will allow your loved one to stay at home longer.

TIP #75

Give to foundations which support research on the disease. Participate in 5K runs or walks. Network with other caregivers. You will constantly leave these events with additional knowledge about the current research on the disease or possible treatment options. You might also realize someone else's current situation may be worse than your own.

HOUSEKEEPING PRAYER

There was a day and a time where families came together ate meals and prayed together. Those days seem long gone and non-existent today. Help us to turn off the television, radio, I-phone and computer and prepare for the future together. It is your desire we prosper and be at peace when "life" happens to us. Help us to communicate better with each other and plan so we are not left in a position where we are hastily making decisions. Allow parents to properly prepare the next generation for the future. Give us the wisdom to obey Habakkuk 2:2 "Write the vision, and make it plain upon tables, that he may run that readeth it." Help us to explain next steps to the next generation that there will be no confusion as to what to do and how to do. We rebuke haphazardness and slothfulness. You said "My people perish for the lack of knowledge." Prepare everyone who reads this book to take necessary preliminary action through proper preparation. In Jesus name. AMEN.

CARE FOR THE CAREGIVER

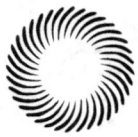

TIP #76

Pick your battles. Family drama could show its ugly head. Your job as a caregiver is one of the hardest jobs there is, if not the hardest. You don't have to fight every battle. Pick and choose your battles.

TIP #77

Being a full-time caregiver for one person is time consuming. However you may have to care for 2 or more. It can significantly interrupt your relationship with the person and, in turn, disturb your own mood and psychological well-being. Their symptoms, level of functioning and perceived happiness will likely trigger symptoms in you. When they are doing well, you will feel relief, at ease and peaceful. When their symptoms are worse, you will feel increased apprehension, depression and overall stress.

But in the midst of it all, pay attention to yourself. You will need to address your needs as well as theirs. Bottling up your frustrations will only cause more frustration. Professional counseling can help you focus and keep things in balance.

TIP #78

If you haven't already, invest in not only term and/or whole life insurance but long term care insurance for yourself as well. We never tend to think it will happen to us, but a sudden illness, injury or unexpected diagnosis can happen to anyone at any time.

The healthier you are right now, the more likely you will live long enough to become frail. During long term care, one would need help with bathing, dressing, eating, toileting, continence, or transferring/moving from a bed to a chair.

Extended care services simply are not fully covered by other types of insurance plans currently available. Disability Insurance does not pay for your care, it only replaces a percentage of lost income. The Affordable Care Act and Medicare does not provide you service for long-term care costs. This is why, as caregivers, we should seriously consider options for private insurance as we ourselves age.

TIP #79

Accept offers of help from others. Be proactive by suggesting things for people to do with the care recipient. Guests should be made aware that coming to visit is not a vacation for them. There is constantly something to be done. Sweeping and mopping the floors, cooking and cleaning and spending quality time with loved ones are good suggestions. Invite guests to come over which do not need to be entertained. They will be your most beneficial asset to both you and the care recipient.

TIP #80

Give yourself credit, treat yourself and pat yourself on the back every now and then for doing the best you can in one of the toughest jobs there is! As a rule of thumb, never wait until everything is perfect before you decide to enjoy your life.

TIP #81

Listen to fellow caregivers talk about their day-to-day experiences through support groups. You may come up with new and effective ideas to lessen your burden. Exchange phone numbers and emails with other caregivers for support.

TIP #82

Turn off the television for extended periods of time. According to research from the School of Population Health at the University of Queensland, Australia, every hour of TV you watch after age 25 cuts your lifespan by 22 minutes.

TIP #83

Be realistic about how much of your time and yourself you can give. Set clear limits, and communicate those limits to doctors, family members, and other people who are involved.

TIP #84

Emotions such as anger, fear, resentment, guilt, helplessness, and grief may show up as a result from your daily caregiving life. For me, it went from anger to frustration to being mad with God and then apologizing and asking God for forgiveness.

It's important to acknowledge and accept what you are feeling. Don't beat yourself up over these emotions. You are human. As an engineer, I often ask *why* and want to know the answers to life's tough questions. I have often asked God these questions:

"Why would you allow me to have ambition and be smart enough to want to finish up a doctorate in a hard core technical field while at the same time be very gifted in serving people through ministry and then care for two parents with radically different needs while I am single all at the same time?

However, I remind myself His strength has given me grace to do it all for so long and therefore I now trust the process. I trust for today as well as for tomorrow.

"Trust in the Lord with all of Thy heart and lean not unto thy own understanding. In all thy ways acknowledge Him and He shall direct thy paths."
Proverbs 3:5-6. (KJV)

TIP #85

Avoid caregiver burnout. Be realistic. Ask yourself these questions:

Can you really work a fulltime job, look after children and care for your ailing loved one simultaneously?

It may be probable or not. Create a to-do list of the tasks you will be responsible for, revise this list often, and avoid being too rigid.

TIP #86

Do things you enjoy that make both you and your loved one happy. Massages for both you and your loved one will help relieve daily stress.

When you need a break to recharge, leave town for a couple of days. Take advantage of any respite program available. Use the Eldercare Locator to find a respite program near you. Go online at www.Eldercare.gov. These are also good times for other family members to help with the caregiving load. I try my best to leave town at least once a month. Going away gives you strength to continue on with the journey.

Pressing the pause button every now and then is a good thing when it comes to caregiving. Everything has a stop at some time or another in order to keep going. To stop, to rest, or to pause means to do nothing. It means no thinking, no moving, and no decisions.

"To make the right choices in life, you have to get in touch with your soul. To do this, you need to experience solitude, which most people are afraid of, because in the silence you hear the truth and not the solutions." (Deepak Chopra)

TIP #87

Exercise regularly. Try to get in at least 30 minutes of exercise at least three times per week. As a caregiver, beware of overeating or lack of exercise. Drastic emotional changes can cause one not to exercise or eat properly. You will eventually find routine exercise relieves stress and gives you energy.

TIP #88

Eat right. Well-nourished bodies are better prepared to cope with stress and get through busy days. Keep your energy up and your mind clear by eating nutritious meals at regular times throughout the day.

TIP #89

Get enough sleep. Aim for an average of eight hours of solid, uninterrupted sleep every night. If you neglect this important process of restoration and renewal only sleep can give, your energy level, productivity, and ability to handle stress will greatly suffer.

TIP #90

As a caregiver, when you rise each morning, there are about 15-20 things to get done before the day ends. Take some quiet time to relax and reflect each morning. Don't beat yourself up for not completing everything. Divide large tasks into smaller tasks over the course of the week or month.

TIP #91

Caregivers have found participating in a support group is a critical lifeline. Support groups allow caregivers to take a break, express concerns, share experiences, and receive emotional comfort. In other words, do not become an island all to yourself. Reach out to family, friends, support groups, counselors and other caregivers for support.

TIP #92

It is okay to say NO. Accept the fact you simply can't do everything! This is especially true when you are not only a caregiver but you have both a very demanding career and are actively involved in your community.

TIP #93

In one year there are 52 weeks, 365 days, 8,765 hours, 525,948 minutes, 31,556,926 seconds of time on your hands. One of those days marks your birthday. Enjoy it and include something special you do for yourself. Birthdays with your loved ones at _Olive Garden_ are quite special.

TIP #94

Keep in mind the care recipients, whether they verbally express it or not, sincerely appreciate the service you provide. They are truly grateful for your daily service. What would their life be without you?

One of the greatest feelings in the world is when someone openly tells you how much you mean to them. This tip says "Thank you" from all care recipients to all caregivers with love.

TIP #95

Read for an hour a day. Reading habits will open up frontiers making you a better producer, a deeper thinker and a richer human. *"A house that has a library in it has a soul."* (Plato)

TIP #96

Rewrite regularly how you would have wished you lived on the last day of your life in your journal. This heightens your focus on doing what counts, and trains your brain to get it done.

TIP #97

Practice removing "complaint" from your vocabulary. Most of the time, complaint is nothing more than frustration and anger.

CAREGIVER'S CARE PRAYER

As caregivers we give up our lives for others. We put dreams and hopes on hold. Our financial income is at an all-time low in most cases. We get little sleep at night and oftentimes we put ourselves last in terms of health and fitness. Give us daily wisdom to put what we cannot solve in Your hands and trust You through the process. Thank You for stretching our faith. In addition to caregiving, You have given some of us the ability to multi-task by having careers and businesses. As we work non-stop, give us wisdom on how to care for ourselves so we can become better equipped to care and work for others. We thank You that You have entrusted, anointed and appointed so great a responsibility on us but we ask that You grace us to use the time wisely. Help us to realize it is okay to say no. Let us be mindful of Matthew 5:37, "But let your communication be, yea, yea; nay, nay. Thank You. In Jesus' name. Amen.

SOCIAL ADVICE

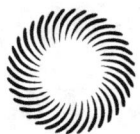

TIP #98

Set specific times when friends can call or text you. As a caregiver your time is very limited. True friends will understand and work around your schedule. A strong friendship doesn't need daily conversation. As long as the relationship lies in the heart, true friends will never part.

TIP #99

Sending cards, texts and flowers to family members and friends are ways one says "I love you" and can make up for a lot of time you simply do not have.

TIP #100

Friends are good resources which help balance your life in positive directions. When you become burned out, pick up the phone and call a friend for a good laugh. Go out to lunch weekly and/or join a book club. You must balance life out with both work and fun. By the way, laughter is regarded as an important antidote to stress.

TIP #101

Your relationships may change while you care for a loved one with Alzheimer's disease. You may not have the time or the energy to do all the things you were used to doing in terms of socializing. Do not take on more responsibility than you possibly can. Again and again, it's okay to say no.

TIP #102

Facebook, Twitter and all other social media outlets are a great way to show friends and relatives which live at a distance pictures of your loved ones. They are also beneficial for communicating. However, remind friends and relatives their cards, calls and visits mean much more to your loved ones, especially if they are not Internet savvy.

TIP #103

Indulge in other activities, whenever the possibility arises, with nearby friends. You both need and deserve some of the pleasures life has to offer.

TIP #104

Caregiving can put a strain on a romantic relationship or marriage. Caregiving can demand more time away from a relationship or marriage, and this can eventually dissolve the relationship. Make sure the two of you discuss and communicate your frustrations. It may take an extra level of trust and commitment to be able to maintain the relationship with a caregiver.

Although I am not married and have never been married, I

have tried dating while caregiving. It has not worked with the demands from caregiving and my career, partly because I consider myself "married" to my career at this time. I can only imagine what life would be within a marriage. I have made the sacrifice and choice to remain single until at least after doctoral work to avoid hurting or being hurt in a relationship.

TIP #105

If you learn to balance and communicate your caregiving duties wisely with your spouse, despite caregiving pressure and demands, you will find deep gratitude and a measure of awe for your spouse's support and understanding. You will ultimately find sharing the experience with a trusted spouse will only strengthen your relationship.

TIP #106

The saying "God will not give us more than we can bear" is not scriptural and is further from truth. The point of living in a fallen world is not for us to try to carry our heavy burdens, but rather surrender them to God so our faith can be stretched. Yes indeed, everything is more than I can handle alone, but not more than Jesus can handle.

"For we do not want you to be unaware, brothers, of the affliction we experienced in Asia. For we were so utterly burdened beyond our strength that we despaired of life itself" **(2 Corinthians 1:8 KJV).** Yet Jesus reminds us to. *"Come to me, all who labor and are heavy laden, and I will give you rest"* **(Matthew 11:28 KJV)**

TIP #107

Philosopher Thomas Aquinas said, *"Friendship is the source of the greatest pleasures, and without friends even the most agreeable pursuits become tedious."* Friends help ease the pain. Many of my friends live outside of the state in which I reside. However when we talk, it gives me strength to endure. Being a lone ranger can make the task overwhelmingly difficult. Support and strength are needed most.

TIP #108

As a caregiver, you will lose friends. Your life as a caregiver will not at all times be understood by everyone. Your time will not always be available for others. You can become a different person in terms of travel, time and social activities.

Small minds cannot comprehend big spirits. In order to be great you must be willing to be mocked, misunderstood, and sometimes hated. Stay strong!

SOCIAL PRAYER

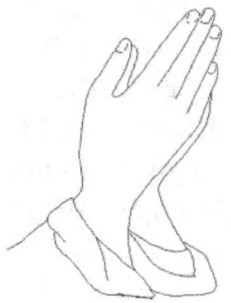

You are our Friend that sticks closer to us than a brother. We thank You for earthly friends. We thank You for opportunities to laugh and confide in friends. Thank You for early morning breakfast or lunch with them. They have been sent to comfort us. Thank You for social media outlets to keep up with them. Thank You for using them as outlets outside of the home. Bless them as they bless us. In Jesus' name. AMEN.

HEALTHY EATING

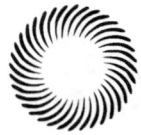

TIP #109

Hippocrates, a Greek physician, once said *"Our food should be our medicine, and our medicine should be our food."*

Being healthy has a lot to do with choosing the right kinds of food to eat. Every time you eat or drink, you are either feeding disease or fighting it. Consult with your physician as well as read the label on anything you eat.

pH levels keep the body healthy and balanced. When we eat foods highly acidic, for example, our body will work to correct it. pH levels are measured on a scale from 0 to 14. Seven is considered neutral; 0 is completely acidic, and 14 is completely alkaline. Your blood needs to be slightly alkaline, with a pH somewhere between 7.35 and 7.45.

TIP #110

Today's modern diet have become high in processed foods. It is both acid-forming and leads to disease and ill health around the globe. Acid-forming foods could lead to kidney and liver damage, potentially even increasing your risk of diabetes.

TIP #111

A study from the Arizona Respiratory Center at the University of Arizona found foods high in acid content (often those with an abundance of animal proteins and salt and low in fruits and vegetables) can lead to "a sub-clinical or low-grade state of metabolic acidosis," potentially leading to an increase in the risk of cancer.

TIP #112

Flavonoids are plant-based nutrients found in fruits and vegetables. Flavonoids offer anti-inflammatory, anti-microbial and anti-oxidative benefits. Examples of foods containing flavonoids are
- Broccoli
- Kale
- Turnip greens
- Spinach
- Blackberries
- Grapes
- Raspberries
- Plums
- Red cabbage
- Lemons
- Grapefruit
- Squash
- Bananas

TIP #113

Saturated fats are linked to heart disease and increase blood cholesterol. Foods from animals such as whole milk, ice cream, cream, cheese, butter, lard and meats are associated with saturated fats. Plant oils such as cocoa butter and palm kernel have saturated fat in them.

TIP #114

Trans-fat is not found naturally in food. It is made when liquid oils are turned solid through hydrogenation. Restaurants and fast-food chains use hydrogenated or partially hydrogenated vegetable oils. Just like saturated fats, trans-fats raise blood cholesterol. Read each food label.

TIP #115

Monounsaturated fats can prevent heart disease and are liquid at room temperature. Plant oils such as olive oil, canola oil and peanut oil are healthy.

TIP #116

Omega-3 fats have been linked to prevention of heart disease, stroke and cancer. Examples are flax seeds, nuts and fish.

TIP #117

Polyunsaturated fats are found in vegetable oil and are liquid at room temperature. Plant oils such as sesame oil, soy oil, corn oil, nuts and seeds are much healthier than saturated fats.

TIP #118

The following words on labels mean they are high in fat, and one should be cautious:

Au beurre, creamy, hollandaise, breaded, scampi, fritters,

batter-dipped, flaky, Alfredo, bisque, crispy, parmigiana, loaded, buttery, flaky

TIP #119

Healthier choices which are lower in fat and calories are: Steamed, baked, grilled, poached, roasted, broiled and boiled.

TIP #120

Choose entrees which feature vegetables, fish, seafood, chicken or lean meat. Decline the bread basket.

TIP #121

If you want salmon and the menu says "salmon with ginger cream", ask if the salmon can be served with "tomato-citrus puree" instead. Be proactive in making special requests.

TIP #122

While preparing food, keep this in mind.
- Reduce sugar by 1/3
- Reduce fat by 1/3
- Omit salt or reduce by ½

TIP #123

Healthy eating habits for both the caregiver and care recipient can prove beneficial to both parties. Work with your physician to determine how much or how little you should consume.

TIP #124

Eating healthy keeps the cells in your body well-nourished and has been known to extend life. A Mediterranean diet is rich in healthy fats (like olive oil), fish, and produce. A study done by the University of Gothenburg showed the chances of living longer increased 20% from eating a Mediterranean diet.

TIP #125

There are several advantages to buying from farmers markets. Their produce is often fresher than grocery produce. They spend less time from picking to eating meaning more nutrients are still present in the food. They spend less time on truck traveling which results in less opportunity for infection by bad bacteria.

TIP #126

The healthiest food to order when you are at a fast-food restaurant includes a veggie burger, mushroom burger, garden salad, English muffin or a baked potato with salsa. You may have to shop around because most fast food outlets do not have this type of food on a menu.

TIP #127

Eat at least two fish meals per week. The oils in darker types of fish, such as salmon, tuna, and herring, are beneficial for both the heart and the brain.

TIP #128

Water is essential and one should drink eight 8-ounce glasses each day. Keep your care recipient well hydrated, especially in warm and humid weather conditions.

TIP #129

Sugar and caffeine should be kept to a minimum. Replace sugar with raw sugar if possible. Sugar is just as harmful as oxidized fats to the body. The chemical structure of sugar contains lots of oxygen molecules and the potential to form reactive bonds. This can result in free radicals. Free radicals are tied to inflammation and the progressive degeneration of any ongoing disease.

TIP #130

Bananas, cantaloupes and oranges are rich in potassium. Eating these may cause one to be less prone to high blood pressure.

TIP #131

Start each day off with breakfast so the body can get the proper carbohydrates it needs. Fruit smoothies are an easy way to nourish your body. There is a "Smoothie King" store I stop in on some mornings. It does my stomach and entire system well. There are a variety of choices. For example, blend strawberries, blueberries, or raspberries with frozen bananas and 100% fruit juice.

TIP #132

It can be difficult to suddenly change eating habits. Eat less from a box and more from the earth. Let us however be mindful of the Holy Scripture,

"Watch and pray, that ye enter not into temptation: the spirit indeed is willing, but the flesh is weak."
Matthew 26:41 (KJV)

HEALTHY EATING PRAYER

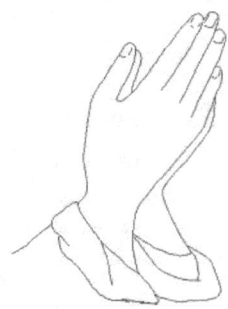

*You have given us our bodies as a temple. You remind us in **1 Corinthians 10:31** "Whether therefore ye eat, or drink, or whatsoever ye do, do all to the glory of God." You are concerned about our food intake and have given the choice to us to decide. You have provided fruit and vegetables from the seed of the ground. We ask You to help us break the cycle of unhealthy eating so that we can live healthier and more productive lives. We know that our bodies live off of proper nutrients. Give us the discipline to heed to Your instruction. Paul reminds us in **1 Corinthians 9:27**, "But I keep under my body, and bring it into subjection: lest that by any means, when I have preached to others, I myself should be a castaway." Give us wisdom from on High and to be mindful of our daily intake. In Jesus' name. AMEN.*

ESSENTIAL OIL BENEFITS

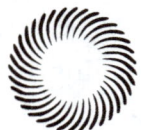

Dear Readers:

You are welcome to purchase essential oils on my website at *www.odellglennessentialoils.com* or at your local store. Wherever you purchase, make sure the essential oil is 100% pure. Through scholarly research, I have proven hinoki, cedar wood and tea tree oil are soluble in both liquid and supercritical carbon dioxide (CO_2). Read more on my website - Thank you.

TIP #133

Essential oils are the purest form of a plant. The liquid out of the plant comes from steam distillation from the plant stems, leaves, flowers, seeds, branches, bark and roots. They date back to 4500 B.C. In 1922, the tomb of King Tut was uncovered. Archeologists found oil in large vases, still as good as the day it was placed in the tomb.

TIP #134

Interest in essential oils has revived in recent decades with the popularity of aromatherapy. Aromatherapy is a branch of alternative medicine which claims essential oils and other aromatic compounds have curative effects.

TIP #135

Even if you are not a Bible believer, essential oils, as proven through scientific research, have shown they may indeed have significant healing effects against bacteria and certain viruses. Further research is still yet to be revealed to its fullest potential. However, the research seems promising.

TIP #136

Researchers from England (2002) found applying lemon balm oil to the faces and arms of patients with severe dementia reduced their agitation by 35 percent.

TIP #137

In 2005, researchers found the scent of lavender increased deep, restful sleep for both men and women.

TIP #138

A research study showed a combination of cedar wood, lavender, rosemary, and thyme oils promoted hair growth among patients with alopecia areata, an autoimmune disorder which causes hair to fall out. Certain blends of oil can prove beneficial.

TIP #139

There are 14 oils mentioned in the Bible:
Myrrh - mentioned 18 times
Frankincense - mentioned 22 times
Calamus (cane) - mentioned 5 times
Cedar wood - mentioned 5 times
Cinnamon - mentioned 4 times
Cassia - mentioned 3 times
Galbanum - mentioned once
Onycha - mentioned once
Spikenard (nard) - mentioned 7 times
Hyssop - mentioned 12 times
Sandalwood (aloes) - mentioned 5 times
Myrtle - mentioned 6 times
Cypress - mentioned once
Rose of Sharon - mentioned once

TIP #140

A few of the more popular aromatic plant oils and their uses for the following symptoms include:

peppermint – digestive disorders

rosemary – muscular pains, mental stimulant

sandalwood – depression, anxiety and nervous tension

sweet orange – depression and anxiety

tea tree – respiratory problems, antifungal, antibacterial and antiviral

lavender – headaches, insomnia, burns, aches and pains.

TIP #141

Essential oils have many properties and are known to be very potent. Some are highly antiseptic and oxygenate cells. Some are disinfectant, raise frequency and remove toxins, poisons and heavy metals. Some oils have been shown to fight viruses, bacteria and even tumors. Apply a few drops of these oils on the bottom of your loved one's feet, behind the ear lobes, around the neck and on the hands.

TIP #142

Peppermint oil has its plant origin in North America, Great Britain and in the Mediterranean. It comes from the botanical family called *lamiacae*. Peppermint is good for digestive orders, headaches, heartburn, insomnia, liver, menstrual cramps, and nervous disorders. It can also be used for rheumatism and arthritis, respiratory infections, obesity, viral infections, fungal infections, and skin conditions. One drop of peppermint oil is equivalent to 26 cups of peppermint tea.

Mom has severe allergies around the spring season. Her usage of peppermint oil has literally shown immediate results.

TIP #143

Frankincense belongs to the botanical family called *burseracae*. It is in the Holy anointing oil used for newborn kings and priests. It helps to reprogram cellular memory which then promotes healing for typhoid, allergies, herpes, tonsilitis, head injuries, depression and cancer.

TIP #144

Myrrh belongs to the same family as Frankincense. Pregnant mothers anointed themselves with myrrh for protection against infectious diseases. Myrrh has a long history for use in skin health and hygiene products and it prolongs the scent of other oils. Myrrh is good to combat wrinkles and is antiseptic, aids in balancing thyroid disease and clears athlete's foot, ringworm, viral hepatitis, inflammation and bronchitis.

TIP #145

Frankincense and myrrh must be crushed and bruised to get the oil out from a tree. Frankincense is a universal oil. Myrrh is a preserver. It was used in biblical times to keep wine from going sour. It was also used to keep the scent of perfumes from fading, and to embalm.

"When they saw the star, they rejoiced with exceeding great joy. And when they were come into the house, they saw the young child with Mary his mother, and fell down, and worshiped him: and when they had opened their treasures, they presented unto him gifts; gold, frankincense, and myrrh."
Matthew 2:11-12 (KJV)

TIP #146

Hyssop was offered to Jesus on the cross. Many think hyssop may have been used to help Him breathe due to its respiratory benefits. The hyssop plant was used during the exodus from Egypt to dab the Hebrews; doorposts with lamb's blood, protecting them from the plague of death.

"Cleanse me with hyssop, and I will be clean; wash me, and I will be whiter than snow."
Psalms 51:7. (KJV)

"A jar of wine vinegar was there, so they soaked a sponge on it, put the sponge on a stalk of hyssop plant, and lifted it to Jesus' lips."
John 19:29 (KJV)

TIP #147

Cedar wood oil is used for skin problems. It is calming and it makes for natural insect repellant. King Solomon built God's temple out of cedar. The Egyptians used it for embalming the dead. Medically, it is used to combat hair loss, acne, tuberculosis and promote mental clarity.

"And he shall take to cleanse the house two birds, and cedar wood and scarlet and hyssop."
Leviticus 14:49 (KJV)

TIP #148

The leaves have essential oils in them. Essential oils refer to "medicine" which help our bodies and heal our ailments.

"Along the bank of the river, on this side and that, will grow all kinds of trees used for food; their leaves will not wither, and their fruit will not fail. They will bear fruit every month, because their water flows from the sanctuary. Their fruit will be for food, and their leaves for medicine."
Ezekiel 47:12 (KJV)

TIP #149

Here again we see the Holy Scriptures referring to the leaves of the tree as healing.

"In the middle of its street, and on either side of the river, was the tree of life, which bore twelve fruits, each tree yielding its fruit every month. The leaves of the tree were for the healing of the nations."
Revelation 22:2 (KJV)

TIP #150

The use of essential oils along with prayer have been used for healing.

"And they cast out many demons, and anointed with oil many who were sick, and healed them."
Mark 6:13 (KJV)

TIP #151

This anointing Mary gave Jesus was in preparation for his death. The essential oil she used was spikenard, a very precious and expensive oil. It is harvested by crushing and bruising the root of the plant to squeeze the oil from it. After this, spikenard was then used for healing. In the same way, Jesus was bruised for our iniquities and our chastisement was on him so our spirits could be healed and given new life.

"Then took Mary a pound of ointment of spikenard, very costly, and anointed the feet of Jesus, and wiped his feet with her hair: and the house was filled with the odor of the ointment."
John 12:3 (KJV)

ESSENTIAL OILS PRAYER

*Y*ou said *"the leaves of the tree were for the healing of the nations." We are aware essential oils are from trees You have provided us here on earth.* We thank You for research discoveries on its potential. We believe You for more proven research. As we use these oils, we open ourselves up to the healing of both body and spirit they provide. In Jesus' name. AMEN.

WHAT "NOT" TO DO AS A CAREGIVER

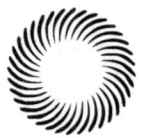

TIP #152

DO NOT pretend you are all the time content and you do not miss the life you had before caregiving. You need time to grieve and miss your old life and time to usher in new norms. Change is not easy.

One of the most humblest moments in the metamorphic process is when caregivers have to sell their own homes or condos and then move in with their loved ones. In addition, to leave and turn down high paying career opportunities and relocate somewhere where you are paid much less than you know you are worth. Your credit score may take a hit.

Furthermore, you may have to relocate with your loved one to a location where your heart is not. Nevertheless, you relocate because it best suits the needs for your loved one. This could ultimately compromise already established relationships.

TIP #153

Your heart will not every time be in it. You will have days in which you will want to be free of the obligation and the commitment. Allow yourself to have "bad" days even though you're doing what needs to be done for the person you care. **DO NOT** feel guilty if resentment arises every now and then. You are made a human being just like everyone else.

To my fellow male caregivers:

DO NOT be afraid to cry. It tends to free your mind from sorrowful thoughts. After you shed some tears, keep hope alive but remembering the Holy Scripture promises joy.

"Weeping may endure for a night, but joy cometh in the morning."
Psalms 30:5 KJV.

TIP #154

DO NOT bottle up your emotions with the person you care for. Of course, every relationship is different, but sharing your struggles with the person you're caring for can make the two of you closer, despite the many changes which occur in both of your daily lives.

TIP #155

DO NOT isolate yourself from other people and social events even if the person you care for is housebound. Life is to be lived to the fullest and you do not want to miss out on other important aspects of your life. Life is too short. Somehow, figure out how to maintain a balanced life in and throughout daily challenges. This may take trial and error efforts but work on it and don't neglect it.

As a caregiver, avoid arguing. If the care recipient does not agree with you, let it be. Arguing usually makes things worse.

TIP #157

DO NOT give up on your dreams and goals. Dating and marriage should not be counted out. Ministerial aspirations should never be pushed aside. Do not leave this world with work undone. Beneath the risk you did not take, lies the dreams which lay dormant. Opportunities will never open up to closed people.

PRAYER ON
WHAT NOT TO DO AS A CAREGIVER

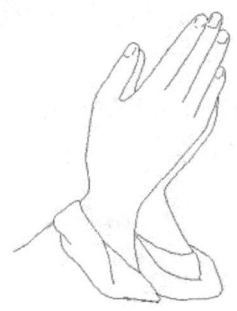

We are human but tend to live extra-human lives. Help us to take care of ourselves emotionally, physically, spiritually, from within, and amid our fellow men. Create such harmony and balance that we radiate Your love through us in all we do and say. Remind us of the lesson between Mary and Martha that we are to always keep ourselves centered on what is most important in life which is serving and loving You. In Jesus' name. AMEN.

BIBLICAL/PHILOSPHICAL PRINCPLES

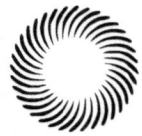

TIP#158

It is more blessed to give than to receive."
Acts 20:3 (KJV).

Periodically send flowers to your loved ones. Allow them to smell the roses while they yet live.

TIP #159

Love is an action word. Observe those who say they "love" you and/or your loved ones. Love denotes "doing" more than "saying." Characterize people by their actions and you will never be fooled by their words.

TIP #160

Remember you were chosen for the assignment. Not everyone can do what God has gifted and given you the strength to do.

"Before I formed thee in the belly I knew thee; and before thou camest forth out of the womb."
Jeremiah 1:5 (KJV)

TIP #161

"Honor thy father and mother; which is the first commandment with promise; that it may be well with thee."
Ephesians 6:2 (KJV)

This Holy Scripture is typically saying as children we have a responsibility for the well-being of parents and guardians.

TIP #162

"Feed the flock of God which is among you, taking the oversight thereof, not by constraint, but willingly; not for filthy lucre, but of a ready mind; Neither as being lords over God's heritage, but being examples to the flock. And when the chief Shepherd shall appear, ye shall receive a crown of glory that fadeth not away."
1 Peter 5:2-4 (KJV)

This Holy Scripture represents care for anyone who you have been entrusted to care for. Lead and care for with a willing heart. Be a good caregiver so others may see your example, and so the care recipient may have confidence in you and become pleased with your work. The Bible tells us there will be a crown waiting which will never fade.

TIP #163

When you become frustrated and feel as if the work you have been given is overwhelmingly difficult, take heed to the Holy Scripture lesson which reminds us to:

"Be strong and of good courage, and do it: fear not, nor be dismayed:

for the LORD *God, even my God, will be with thee; he will not fail thee, nor forsake thee, until thou hast finished all the work for the service of the house of the* LORD.*"*
1 Chronicles 28:20 (KJV)

When everyone and everything around you seems as if it is failing, God will not. The work He has begun through you will be finished through His grace. The work you are doing is for His house. Dedicate your house to God and watch Him protect, guide and direct.

TIP #164

"Trust in the Lord with all your heart and lean not on your own understanding; in all your ways acknowledge him and he will direct your path."
Proverbs 3:5–6 (KJV)

I cannot emphasize enough the importance of asking God for His wisdom and guidance each and every day. After you do this, trust Him to help you make the best decisions. Each day is different and comes with different challenges, but He will be faithful if you allow Him to.

TIP #165

"The light of the eyes rejoiceth the heart: and a good report maketh the bones fat."
Proverbs 15:30 (KJV).

The facts may say there is no known cure, and each day you

may witness the deterioration of your loved one, but a smile, a joke, a laugh, a hug each day does indeed bring back life. Make sure your home has some joy in it.

TIP #166

"I will lift up mine eyes unto the hills, from whence cometh my help. My help cometh from the LORD, which made heaven and earth."
Psalms 121:1-2(KJV)

There are days, weeks, moments, and sometimes seasons where everyone seems busy. Your life and everything around you looks disordered, the funds have dried up, and you feel desolate and alone.

The doctors and nurses have no answers but advise things may worsen, your research and career is not going smoothly, your peers do not understand you, your friends are few, and your family may have deserted you or have secretly desired you to fail.

When you are going through a wilderness-type experience like this, lift your eyes toward your help. There is help and it comes from above. This is where you will have to use earlier tips and rest, relax, read a book or go away to get your strength. There will indeed be seasons like this, but balance is key. He made the Heavens and Earth, so He can certainly tend to your household.

TIP #167

"I will both lay me down in peace, and sleep."
Psalms 4:8 (KJV).

At all times try and get a peaceful sleep. Even if you have

to hire another caregiver to watch over your loved one while you get an 8-hour night of rest, peace and sleep. Try to do it, for you cannot be your best without it.

TIP #168

"He giveth power to the faint; and to them that have no might he increaseth strength."
Isaiah 40:29 (KJV)

Many questions asked of me, "How do you do and accomplish so much with very little help?" My first response is my help comes from above. My prayer each day is not to possess homes, cars and material things. It is for daily guidance and wisdom. Secondly, it is He that gives me the strength and grace to do all I do. When I am weak, He lifts me. There are many days when I am at the end of patience, but He comes in and gives me more strength. I cannot explain how He does it but He is faithful each and every time.

TIP # 169

"Give, and it shall be given unto you; good measure, pressed down, and shaken together, and running over, shall men give into your bosom. For with the same measure that ye mete withal it shall be measured to you again."
Luke 6:38 (KJV)

As you give your time and service to caregiving, you will find you will lack nothing. Most caregivers I talk with have no real needs other than the need for more hands to help for the task before them. Jesus reminded us the "Harvest is ripe, but the laborers are few." The world teaches us to hoard things up for ourselves and "do you." But as you give, it shall be given to you. You won't have to worry about who or how you will be taken care of once you grow old. The earth gives what you give to it.

TIP #170

> *"Casting all your care upon him; for He careth for you."*
> **1 Peter 5:7 (KJV)**

When I get older, who will look after me? Will I ever make the money I used to make? Will the dreams and goals I once had ever come to be? Will I marry or will I grow old alone? Can I dream again? Will things ever get better? Will my child put me in an assisted living home? Will my children and grandchildren ever come to visit me? Will holidays be lonely?

These are questions caregivers often ask themselves as they think about the future. Most of us have put our careers, relationships and finances on hold to give care full-time. The Holy Scripture is encouraging by emphasizing we have someone who cares for us. We must cast these questions and concerns on Him and believe Him to finish the work He began in us.

TIP #171

> *"For the LORD seeth not as man seeth; for man looketh on the outward appearance, but the LORD looketh on the heart."*
> **1 Samuel 16:7 (KJV)**

People may judge you from the outside, but they do not know who you are and whose you are. The Holy Scripture reminds us

God sees your heart. When you give care willingly, God sees and will reward you. When someone has your heart, there is pure genuine love around you. People who judge you do not know your heart and in most cases don't have compassion for your loved ones either. Pray for wisdom and you will know who they are.

"It's 3 a.m. and I have not slept 4 hours in 3 days!! I have a family of 10 and no one has come to offer any help!!"

"After all the free food and lodging my loved one gave, very few have even picked up the telephone to call!! Is it true once one gets old, folks forget you? Lord, I'm afraid!"

"My loved one has been in the hospital for 3 days and no one has come to visit?! Why, God, why?"

"My own health is failing, but how can I see a doctor and monitor my health when my loved one's health is worse? I'm crying, depressed and sad and no one seems to care."

"I've prayed, I've fasted, I've gone to every church service I know but I'm in the same situation. Lord, I need your help."

TIP #172

"For I reckon that the sufferings of this present time are not worthy to be compared with the glory which shall be revealed in us."
Romans 8:18 (KJV)

Caregivers smile but internally they cry. Paul reminds us this type of suffering is nothing compared to the glory. Jesus suffered on the cross for us, but three days later He arose. As we go through these experiences, allow God's glory to show through you. Trust me, it will be okay. These are those very times you exercise your faith muscles. Storms make you strong and mature you as a believer. Sometimes, God gives us a hard assignment and some questionable requirements, however He gives us the strength to endure through wilderness experiences. Trust the process. You will gain more from going through than not.

Big hugs from me to you!!!

TIP #173

"But the fruit of the Spirit is love, joy, peace, longsuffering, gentleness, goodness, faith."
Galatians 5:22 (KJV)

We do not talk much of it, but longsuffering, is a part of the fruit of the Spirit. Suffering grows strength. Your trials and tribulations can indeed serve your growth. Pain today can leverage into greater humility, bravery and love later on.

Longsuffering, along with patience, love, gentleness, goodness and faith are all of the characteristics of a caregiver. Let us safely say caregiving is a daily job which demonstrates all of the fruits of the Spirit. You are truly special in God's eyesight.

TIP #174

"Speak up for those who cannot speak for themselves, for the rights of all who are destitute, speak up and judge fairly; defend the rights of the poor and needy."
Proverbs 31:8-9

Protest, run, march, picket, vote and write to Congress for the elderly and for those like you who are caregivers. Make your vote count by voting for protection and funds for further research on the disease as well as funds will that would help you as caregiver. Never allow anyone to take advantage of your loved ones.

TIP #175

"Thou hast turned for me my mourning into dancing: thou hast put off my sackcloth, and girded me with gladness; To the end that my glory may sing praise to thee, and not be silent. O LORD my God, I will give thanks unto thee forever."
Psalms 30:11-12 (KJV)

Each day is a blessing as you and your loved one wake up to see a brand new day together. Whenever your loved one smiles or laughs with you, praise God and thank Him for it. Sing songs of praise. It is a blessing to turn sadness into joy and dancing. You will be surprised at the results.

TIP #176

"Verily I say unto you, Inasmuch as ye have done it unto one of the least of these my brethren, ye have done it unto me."
Matthew 25:40 (KJV)

As caregivers, you already know not many people will ever stop by to visit your home, the nursing facility or the hospital. The poor, needy and helpless often seem overlooked. But know someone is watching you. Your heart will sometimes hurt in pain through this level of service, but constantly remind yourself you are actually serving God. Rejoice in knowing your labor is not in vain.

TIP #177

Philosopher CH. Lewis said *"Hardship often prepares an ordinary person for an extraordinary destiny."* Hardship prepares you for greatness. It opens the door and allows for opportunities for you to teach life's hard lessons to others. You never know where you will end up after a difficult journey but you can be assured you will have grown as a person.

TIP #178

Aristotle said *"We are what we repeatedly do. Greatness then is not an act, but a habit."*

Year after year, day after day, week after week, hour after hour, second after second caregiving becomes who you are You are wiser than you were the day before. Your faith grows stronger each year. You become more skilled than you were last year. You become more confident, and the love you give becomes greater than it was before. Your habits will hopefully become contagious.

TIP #179

Philosopher Crissy Jami said, *"Christianity, like genius, is one of the hardest concepts to forgive. We hear what we want to hear and accept what we want to accept, for the most part, simply because there is nothing more offensive than feeling like you have to re-evaluate your own train of thought and purpose in life. You have to die to an extent in your hunger for faith, for wisdom, and quite frankly, most people aren't ready to die."*

Faith is unforeseen and so it becomes a denial of self. In our society, we are taught to believe what we see and not focus on what will be. Our churches have become entertainment-oriented and reality television has become the fad of the day. This is the very reason why caregivers are far and in between. It is not a popular, gratifying job. It requires one to stretch faith. It requires work which many are not willing to do. Most people simply want a life of convenience to fulfill self-gratification.

TIP #180

Philosopher Cody McGuire said *"Be as good as you can be; there you will find happiness."* As a caregiver, when you have done your utmost best for the day, there is a sense of contentment within you which gives you peace. Live in that moment.

TIP #181

Philosopher Chris Prentis said, *"There is only one way to achieve lasting happiness. That is simply: Be happy."* The Bible tells us to

"Choose ye this day." This tells us we have a choice in the matter. We can choose to be happy and smile each day or we can choose to be sad and depressed for long periods of time. There are ways to live around daily moods. Find the good in each moment and you will find out there are more good and happy moments than sad and disappointing ones. Take time out to count your blessings.

TIP #182

The hours ordinary people waste, extraordinary people leverage. You are extraordinary in every sense of the word, and your time is limited and valuable. Keep in mind time is a precious commodity.

TIP #183

Just because you could not do something yesterday does not mean you cannot achieve it today. You are one day stronger today. Holy Scripture tells us in **Philippians 4:13 (KJV)** *"I can do all things through Christ."* Never settle for anything but the best.

TIP #184

The beautiful thing about "fear" is when you run toward it, it runs away. Fear is false evidence appearing real. When we learn to conquer our fears, then and only then will we begin to see what it really is.

TIP #185

To uplift others when you least feel like it is to join the ranks of the heroic. You are a hero in so many ways to so many people. "Takers" do not inspire the world. However "givers," like yourself, do each day.

BIBLICAL/PHILOSOPICAL PRAYER

You remind us to "be careful for nothing; but in everything by prayer and supplication with thanksgiving let our requests be made known unto God." Your Word gives us hope each day for the challenge. We are content as we meditate and believe on Your Word. They give us life. You love us and are concerned about our daily endeavors. For that, we thank You. "Because thy loving kindness is better than life, our lips will praise You." You left us with Psalms 91:1 that encourages our hearts that if we dwell in the secret place of the most High, we shall abide under the shadow of Your Almighty hands. We acknowledge You in all we do or say. Thank You for constant reminders of Your promises. We lean and trust on Your Word, for it is quick and powerful and sharper than any two-edged sword." Thank You for each promise. We believe and receive. In Jesus' name. AMEN.

CAREGIVER REWARDS

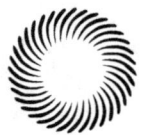

TIP#186

Knowledge + Experience = Wisdom. I have combined a plethora of degrees, experiences and God given gifts into one conglomerate entity. My mantra is to serve people through my knowledge base. Add your caregiving experiences and skills as a pathway to disseminate information in your genre.

"If you cannot figure out your purpose, figure out your passion. For your passion will lead you right into your purpose."
(T.D. Jakes)

The things you are passionate about are not random, they are your calling. Once you figure out what you are passionate about, be so good at what you do others cannot take their eyes or mouth off of you. Life, at times, is about risking everything for a dream no one can see but yourself. I found my voice and discovered my purpose. All along my purpose was attached to my passion.

TIP #187

See your work as your craft. Devote yourself to knowing more about what you do than anyone who has ever done what you do. Follow up on best caregiving techniques through reading and attending group discussions. Learn from others. You will know you have mastered a skill when you are able to teach someone else.

In my secular profession, I am constantly inspiring others. Similarly as a caregiver, your accomplishments are meaningless unless you are inspiring others to set goals at levels higher and better than what you have already done.

TIP #188

A genius is usually misunderstood before they are revered. Taking risks is a step of faith, especially when you are gifted at several things. Do not be surprised by being misunderstood by others. If people aren't laughing at your dreams, your dreams are probably not big enough.

I personally consider myself a simple person with a complicated mind. The movie "A Beautiful Mind", an American biographical film on the life of John Nash is currently my favorite movie.

You dishonor yourself whenever you play small with your full potential. A friendly reminder: you were born into genius. At any age and within any given time frame can you tap into your genius and move from potential to great. You may realize your genius at any age so do not be too concerned if it is yet to emerge at an age which is not considered the norm.

TIP #189

Our minds are shaped from the books we read. Our character is shaped from the people we meet. Our spirit is shaped from the love we give. As caregivers, we give out selfless love each day. In turn, we are daily shaping our spirit.

TIP #190

The moment we decide to give up on our dreams is the moment we die while we yet live. I do not care how young or how old of a caregiver you are; never give up on traveling to the places you want to visit, the degrees you want to obtain, the location you want to live in and the desires of your heart. Run towards them instead of running away from them. It is better to be an optimist who gets disappointed than a pessimist who has no hope.

TIP #191

The best classroom in the world is at the foot of an elderly person. Your time, talent and service as a full-time caregiver are worth every second given each and every year to them. Accept what is, let go of what was, and have faith in what will be.

TIP #192

Caregiving includes a sense of giving back to someone who has previously cared for you.

TIP #193

Caregiving involves the satisfaction of knowing your loved one is getting excellent care.

TIP #194

Caregiving integrates a caregiver's own personal growth and increases meaning and understanding of one's own purpose in life. Life as a caregiver is happening "for" you and not "to" you. Opportunities present themselves when you prepare and give it your all. When it's all said and done, you want to be able to say you've done your best and be at peace with yourself.

TIP #195

You wake up every day to new challenges. You keep going. Why? Because you care! You give up your life to care for another which essentially is the ultimate act of love. Caregiving involves selfless, noble and generous actions directly from the heart.

TIP #196

There are several positive benefits from caregiving. Among them is a wholesome relationship with the care recipient. You both learn a lot from each other. Another aspect is a sense of value and self-esteem one develops from daily care. This develops into instant satisfaction.

TIP#197

A positive aspect of caregiving is being at peace with yourself and with the loved one under your watch. You are assured they are being treated fairly and with respect.

TIP #198

"To everything there is a season, and a time to every purpose under the heaven: A time to be born... a time to plant, a time to heal...a time to build up....a time to laugh.... a time to dance...and a time to love."
Ecclesiastes 3:1 (KJV)

Enjoy each moment while you have the chance!!!

TIP #199

When you are in the valley of pain, take the time to search your heart and look for the growth of the experience. Learning from the growth is how you will eventually rise to the mountaintop.

While caregiving, you will find your hardest times will often lead you to your greatest moments. Keep the faith. It will all be worth it in the end. By yourself, you will never be able to calm the storm, but what you can do is calm yourself. Storms will pass over. The life of a caregiver "is what it is." At the end of the day, there is a peace in knowing you have done your best to make your loved one's day a little brighter.

TIP #200

Just as gravity pulls objects to the center of the earth, there is also a law for sowing and reaping. As you sow in love and care, you will soon reap a harvest.

"And let us not be weary in well doing: for in due season we shall reap, if we faint not."
Galatians 6:9 (KJV)

CAREGIVING REWARDS PRAYER

We realize You have anointed us for this specific work. We are confident You have begun a good work in us and will perform it until the day of Christ Jesus. We give our gifts back to You and are available to be used by You. Use us in the marketplace, in schools, churches, hospitals, supermarkets and wherever You have destined our feet to land. We thank You in advance. In Jesus' name. AMEN.

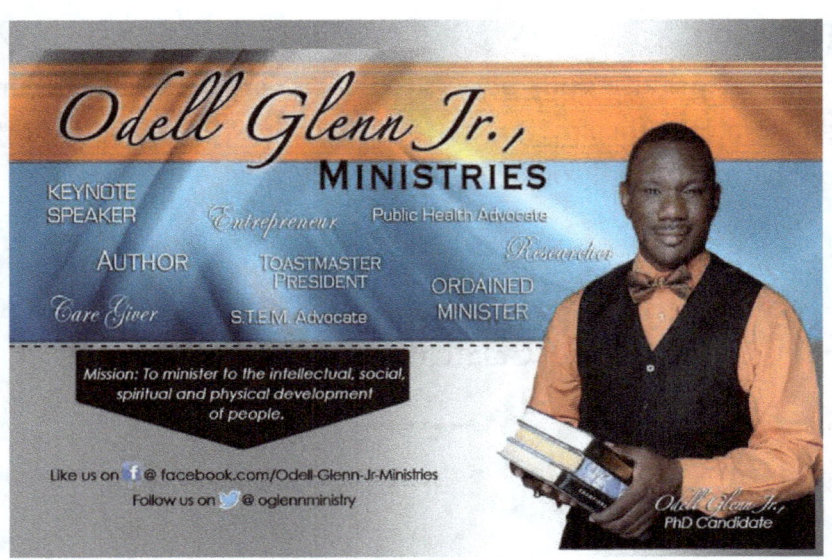

The Lord bless you and keep you; the LORD make His face shine on you, And be gracious to you ; the LORD lift up his countenance on you, And give you peace.
Numbers 6:24-26 (KJV)

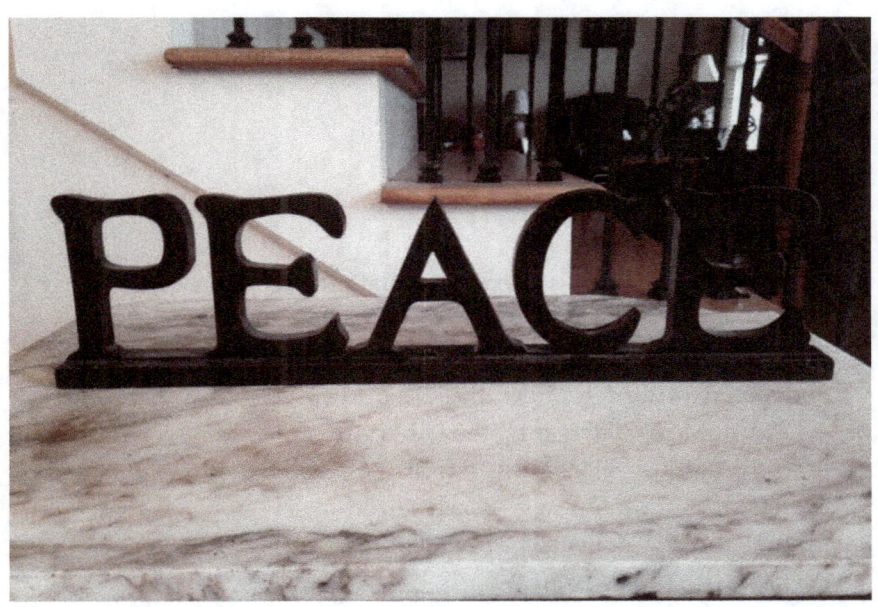

REFERENCES

In reference to: The position of the children of the aging in relation to their parents, children, and grandchildren exposes them to a unique set of unshared stresses in which giving of resources and service far outweighs receiving or exchanging them.

Source: Miller, Dorothy A. "The 'sandwich' generation: adult children of the aging." Social Work (1981) 26 (5): 419-423. doi: 10.1093/sw/26.5.419.

Link: Oxfordjournals.org

In reference to: There is a sense of isolation felt
By millions of unpaid individuals who provide the
bulk of long-term care.
Source: Edward Alan Miller, Susan M. Allen
& Vincent Mor: "Navigating the Labyrinth of
Long-Term Care: Shoring Up Informal Caregiving
in a Home and Community-Based World."
Journal of Aging & Social Policy (2008) 21(5)
Link: Tandfonline.com

In reference to: A striking increase was found (from 34.9% to 52.8%) in the proportion of primary caregivers working alone, without secondary caregiver involvement.

Source: Jennifer L. Wolff, PhD and Judith D. Kasper, PhD: "Caregivers of Frail Elders: Updating a National Profile." The Gerontologist", Copyright by the Gerontological Society of America (2006): 46(3): pages 344-356

Link: **Gerontologist.oxfordjournals.com**

In reference to: A reported 37% of caregivers quit their jobs or reduced their work hours to care for someone age 50+ in 2007.
Source: AARP Public Policy Institute 2008: "*Valuing the Invaluable: The Economic Value of Family Caregiving.*"
Link: **assets.aarp.org**

In reference to: Caregivers also frequently have interrupted sleep, especially for those taking care of dementia patients who may wander or have other needs at night.

Source: Jeanne Alongi and Maggie Moore.
"CDC Seeks to Protect Health of Family Caregivers." NAC, 2006: National Alliance for Caregiving, Evercare Study of Caregivers in Decline, 2006.
Link: **healthy aging critical issues brief**

In reference to: Prayer is the key and faith unlocks the door.
Source: NAC, 2004: National Alliance for Caregiving/AARP, "Caregiving in the U.S.", 2004.
Link: **us caregiving**

In reference to: Women are more likely to help with housework and prepare meals than men.

Source: NAC, 2004: National Alliance for Caregiving/AARP, "Caregiving in the U.S", 2004.
Link: Caregiving in the U.S.

In reference to: Research suggests the number of male caregivers may be increasing and will continue to do so due to a variety of social demographic factors.
Source: *[Kramer, B. J. & E. H. Thompson, (eds.), "Men as Caregivers", (New York: Prometheus Books, 2002). Also "More Men Take on Caregiver Role" by* Karina Bland, (The Arizona Republic June 23, 2013)
Link: Men in Caregiver Role

In reference to: Those who volunteered for two or more organizations experienced a 63% lower likelihood of dying during the study period.
Source: Stephen G. Post, "Altruism, happiness, and health: it's good to be good" International Journal of Behavioral Medicine. (2005): 12(2): pages 66-77.
Link: Altruism happiness and health

In reference to: Watching television for 6 hours a day can cut your life expectancy down by five years.
Source: By Amanda Chan, Huffington Post. "1 Hour Of TV Could Shorten Your Lifespan: Study."

Link: 1 Hour of TV

In reference to: A high consumption of red meat was related to higher all-cause mortality.

Source: Sabine Rohrmann, Kim Overvad and H Bas Bueno-de-Mesquita. BMC Medicine. "Meat consumption and mortality - results from the European Prospective Investigation into Cancer and Nutrition. *BMC Medicine* 2013, 11:63 doi:10.1186/1741-7015-11-63

Link: Meat consumption

In reference to: Diet-induced acidosis may influence molecular activities at the cellular level promote carcinogenesis or tumor progression.

Source: Ian Forrest Robey: *"Examining the relationship between diet-induced acidosis and cancer."* Nutrition & Metabolism (London) 2012 August 1; 9(1):72. doi: 10.1186/1743-7075-9-72.

Link: Nutrition & Metabolism

In reference to: Research studies ever since the 1950s have shown a Mediterranean diet, based on a high consumption of fish and vegetables and a low consumption of animal-based products such as meat and milk, leads to better health.

Source: University of Gothenburg. "Mediterranean diet gives longer life", Swedish study suggests, Science Daily, 20 December 2011

Link: Mediterranean diet

In reference to: Labels which are high in fat. Healthier choices which are low in fat. Salmon with ginger cream should be replaced with tomato-citrus puree. Things to keep in mind while preparing food. Advantages in buying from farmer's markets over regular supermarkets. Fruit which are rich in potassium. The healthiest things to order while at a fast-food restaurant. Two fish meals per week. Sugar and caffeine kept at minimum.

Source: University of South Carolina. "Healthy Eating And Active Living in the Spirit. (HEALS) Participant Manual. Face for Change."

Link: Nutrition & Metabolism

In reference to: Over the past few years a number of clinical trials have compared aromatherapy, principally using either lavender (Lavandula angustifolia or Lavandula officinalis) or lemon balm (Melissa officinalis), with inactive treatment. All of these studies demonstrated a significant impact on behavioral problems in patients with dementia, with negligible side-effects. However, there is still not sufficient evidence to recommend widespread use in clinical practice.

Source: Holmes C., & Ballard, C. "Aromatherapy in dementia" Advances in Psychiatric Treatment Jun 2004, 10 (4) 296-300; DOI: 10.1192/apt.10.4.296

Link: Aromatherapy in dementia

In reference to: Lavender increased the percentage of deep or slow-wave sleep (SWS) in men and women.

Source: Goel,N., Kim Hyungsoo, Lao, R. "An Olfactory Stimulus Modifies Nighttime Sleep in Young Men and Women." 10.1080/07420520500263276, pages 889-904

Link: Nighttime sleep in young men and women

In reference to: The hours ordinary people waste, extraordinary people leverage. To uplift others when you least feel like it is to join the ranks of the heroic. Be so good at what you do that others cannot take their eyes or mouth off of you. See your work as your craft. Our minds are shaped from the books we read. The moment we decide to give up on our dreams is the moment we die. It is better to be an optimist who gets disappointed than a pessimist who has no hope. Accept what is, let go of what was and have faith in what will be.

Source: Sharma, Robin. "Helping People in Organizations Lead

without a title."
Link: http://www.robinsharma.com/

In reference to: In multiple tips citing Holy Scriptures.
Source: Authorized version King James Bible (KJV)
Link: King James Bible online

SPECIAL THANKS

If I had 1000 tongues, I would not be able to say thanks enough to my Lord and Savior Jesus Christ. My life continues to be touched by both Your Presence and Your Spirit. Through faith, hope, trust and belief, I have seen and continue to see Your handiwork in and throughout this labyrinth called life. Thank You for grace which continues to carry me along the journey. I am traveling the road less traveled but am aware and rejoice in the fact You have ordained me for this very path.

Whether it was a prayer, a kind act, a smile, a telephone call, a concern, an email, a text, an instant message, a card or hug, that made the road for both me and my family a little brighter, I sincerely thank, appreciate and love each of you from the depth of my heart.

6 a.m-6:30 a.m. prayer ministry team / Saturday morning mall prayer walks
Siblings: Kermit Glenn and Xanthus Jacobs
The Glenn family and friends
The Ables family and friends
The Campbell family and friends
The Hopkins family and friends
The Peterson family and friends
The Swain family and friends
The Raiford family and friends
The Dean family and friends
The Stevens family and friends
The Means family and friends
The Norris family and friends
The Coleman family and friends
The Stroman family and friends
The Gantt family and friends
The Jacobs family and friends
The Foster family and friends
The Watson family and friends
The LaFrance family and friends
The Pinnock family and friends
All of my personal friends
All of Mom and Dad's personal friends
Social media friends and acquaintances
Kingdom Builders Publications, LLC
Mike Takieddine, Content Editor
All of my book reviewers for your honest opinion

The Scarborough Parish Community
Every caregiver paid or unpaid that has and ever will come to offer help
All beauticians, barbers, photographers, nail and feet salons which have serviced us
Derrick Chiles- my personal barber
Great Clips in Lexington, South Carolina
ReneLuvNCare Caregiving Services
Photographer – Aldrick Williams, Atlanta, Georgia
Photographer and make-up artist – Bobby Thornton, Atlanta, Georgia
Photographer – Scott Krause, Columbia, South Carolina
Photographer – Lashanda Howard, Columbia, South Carolina
Xy-Fy Fotography – New York, New York
J.C. Penney Photo Shoots West Columbia, South Carolina
Hampton Inn, Lexington, South Carolina
The Jefferson Avenue Block Association, Brooklyn, New York
Horace E. Greene Day Care Center, Brooklyn, New York
Hebron Baptist Church and Outreach Ministry, Brooklyn, New York
Universal Baptist Church, Brooklyn, New York
Pilgrim Church and Bishop Donald Oliver, Brooklyn, New York
Universal Temple Church of God, Brooklyn, New York
New Greater Bethel Ministries and Minister Annette Washington, Queens, New York
Zoe Ministries, New York, New York
The Greater Allen A.M.E. Cathedral of New York
Mt. Nebo Full Gospel Baptist Church, Bridgeport, Connecticut
Walking with Jesus Ministries and Pastor Wade, Bridgeport, Connecticut
Mount Olive Church of God in Christ, New Britain, Connecticut
Liberty Christian Center International, Hartford, Connecticut
Prayer and Praise Fellowship, Inc, Hartford, Connecticut
Lexington Senior Center, Lexington, South Carolina
Lexington Interfaith Community Services (LICS), Lexington, South Carolina
The entire staff at Palmetto Senior Care, Cayce, South Carolina
The caregiver's support group at Palmetto Senior Care, West Columbia, South Carolina
The entire staff at Aiken Regional Medical Center Hospital, Aiken, South Carolina
The entire staff at Heartland of Lexington Rehabilitation, West Columbia, South Carolina
The entire staff at Palmetto Health Richland, Columbia, South Carolina
The entire staff at Palmetto Surgery Center, Columbia, South Carolina
The entire staff at Pruitt Health-Columbia in Columbia, South Carolina
The entire staff at Lexington Medical Center Extended Care in Lexington, South Carolina
Lexington Baptist Church Counseling Center, Lexington, South Carolina
The University of South Carolina Counseling Center, Columbia, South Carolina
St. Johns All Nations Church of God in Christ, Portland, Oregon
Superintendent Cliff Chappell
Destiny Church/ Global Impact Group and Pastors John and China Cleveland, California based

Calvary Baptist Church, Lexington, South Carolina
Universal Outreach Church of God in Christ, Irmo, South Carolina
Superintendent Alonzo Johnson, friends and 6 a.m. prayer team
South Carolina Church of God in Christ Jurisdiction, St. Matthews, South Carolina
St. Noah Church of God in Christ, Aiken, South Carolina
New Bethel A.M.E. Church, Lexington, South Carolina
7th Episcopal District of the AME Church
New Bethel A.M.E. noon day prayer team
Brookland Baptist Church, West Columbia, South Carolina
Greater Works Church, Asheville, North Carolina
Superintendent Ronald Gates
University City Church, Charlotte, North Carolina
Covenant Churches and Ministries International
Bishop A. Stevens and Evangelist Stevens
Mother Beverly DeJournett
Mt. Alpha Baptist Church, Ward, South Carolina
Ridge Hill Baptist Church, Ridge Spring, South Carolina
The entire staff at Bright Star Senior Home Care Center, Lexington, South Carolina
Dr. Conigliaro Jones and entire staff at TLM Medical Services
Dr. Alric C. Blake and entire staff at Carolina Vision Center
Dr. Scott Thompson and entire staff at Carolina Eye, Nose and Throat
Haute Choc'lat Multimedia Group
Patrice Delk and Mi Jo Consulting
Manchester Community College, Manchester, Connecticut
College of Technology (COT) and Regional Center for Next Generation Manufacturing (RCNGM), Farmington, Connecticut
Oregon State University, Department of Chemical Engineering, Corvallis, Oregon
Lexington High School, Lexington, South Carolina
Midlands Technical Community College, Columbia, South Carolina
Dr. Ed Gatzke, Toastmasters Founder at the University of South Carolina-Columbia. Special thanks for the University of South Carolina Toastmasters Community for public speaking opportunities to present these tips before publishing
Payne Theological Seminary, Wilberforce, Ohio
University of South Carolina-Columbia, Department of Chemical Engineering; Special thanks to my advisor, Dr. Michael A. Matthews, The Dense Phase Fluids Laboratory Team and the Carbo Nix company
Tyler Evans at the University of South Carolina-Columbia writing center. Thanks for providing free editing service to me as a
graduate student at USC

MORE ABOUT THE AUTHOR
HOW I BECAME A CAREGIVER

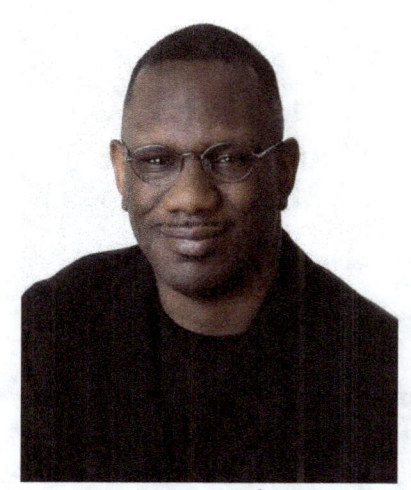

I was at a conference in Hawaii when I received the phone call from my father that my sister passed away in the hospital. My parents were getting older and this, of course, devastated the entire family. In the interim, my dad started to lose memory alongside hip problems. My mom, although relatively healthy at the time was getting older and needed help.

While this drastic life event took place, I was in the prime of my career as an assistant professor at a community college and had decided to embark full time on doctoral work. I had already gotten acceptance packages from several major universities across the country. Simultaneously, my ministerial career reached a plateau as I was also asked to pastor a church.

After evaluating the circumstances, with other siblings living outside of the vicinity from where my parents lived, I decided not to accept any of it and chose to put it all on hold to become a caregiver for my parents.

This involved several relocations and life adjustments. I have been caregiving full-time since June of 2007 after eulogizing my own sister's funeral. Every year has had its challenges, inclusive of falls, hip replacements, surgeries, operations and juggling three schedules. Nevertheless, after 8 years, through the grace of God, I am completing my PhD, am ordained, have my own ministry and am caregiving full-time. I have learned how to integrate caregiving into my life and keep my life moving forward to fulfill His destiny.

Caregiving is indeed unchartered territory and one's emotions run rampant. I have never married nor have children, but it is quite evident I am married to my current lifestyle at this time with little to no room for anything else at the moment. I took on the responsibility of caregiving with no reader's guide and very little, if any, advice. Experience has been my hardest teacher. It gave me the test first and the lesson afterward. I did my work. Now, through this work, I serve as a model for you to do yours. My book is thus intended to help caregivers navigate the journey with guidelines. Many times our trials reveal how God wants us to help others. This work is intended to give the caregiver a framework from which to live each day. The book allows one moments to reflect, smile, vent and/or cry.

Everyone will have its own unique caregiving dilemma. Put simply, caregiving is defined as the very act of serving selflessly from the heart. My hope and prayer is for these tips to inspire, encourage and inform you along your journey. The book also serves as a guide for those who will be caregivers at some point in the future. Prayers have been provided throughout the book. My prayers are continual for both you and your care recipient(s). Grace, mercy and peace be multiplied unto each of you and your families every day and all day!

www.ingramcontent.com/pod-product-compliance
Lightning Source LLC
Chambersburg PA
CBHW072053290426
44110CB00014B/1665